SLEEP BETTER BABY

Thorsons
An imprint of HarperCollins*Publishers*
1 London Bridge Street
London SE1 9GF
www.harpercollins.co.uk
HarperCollins*Publishers*
1st Floor, Watermarque Building, Ringsend Road
Dublin 4, Ireland

First published by Thorsons 2022

3 5 7 9 10 8 6 4 2

A catalogue record of this book is available from the British Library

ISBN 978-0-00-855515-3

Printed and bound in the UK using 100% renewable electricity at CPI Group (UK) Ltd

MIX
Paper | Supporting responsible forestry
FSC
www.fsc.org
FSC™ C007454

This book is produced from independently certified FSC™ paper to ensure responsible forest management.

For more information visit: www.harpercollins.co.uk/green

SLEEP BETTER BABY

The Essential Stress-free Guide to Sleep for You and Your Baby

CAT CUBIE & SARAH CARPENTER

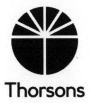

Thorsons

Indy, Roar and Ever – this book couldn't have been written without you ... (and at times it was pretty hard to write it with you!).
Love you always. CC

Harry, Alfie and Emily, I couldn't have done it without your support and understanding that mummy's job isn't 9–5. Now we can go back to bedtime stories. Love you. SC x

Contents

Part III: The Sleep Mums' Routines

Contents

Foreword

'Babies don't come with a manual.'

As Cat and Sarah say, this is a joke that is often cracked but isn't funny. It never helps frazzled parents who are struggling to understand the language of their new baby, loving their baby with every piece of themselves, yet longing for a night's sleep.

So, thank goodness for Cat and Sarah, aka The Sleep Mums. They have not written a manual. They understand that each baby is unique, that one size will not fit all and that parents need safe, sensible advice delivered in a non-judgmental way.

The Sleep Mums have done SO much more than write a manual. They have constructed a very simple framework around which parents can build their own schedule, to find a routine that works for them and their families.

In the dark days of the Covid-19 pandemic, when new parents were literally all alone in isolation, their chirpy voices streamed out from their award-winning podcast. This podcast was kind in tone, broad-ranging and groundbreaking. The Sleep Mums brought solace and wisdom to countless parents in the silence of lockdown. Their podcast could not be equalled.

Until now.

Quietly, in the background, Cat and Sarah were bringing their huge, combined experience to bear on a book. Cat has a degree in psychology, so she understands people on a whole different level. Sarah started her career as a Norland Nanny and went on to develop her own sleep-consultancy practice, which she has run for 20 years. Between them, they have six young children, so not only do they have the smarts, they have also done the hard graft.

And so, this book was born. I have read it, cover to cover. And despite being a paediatrician with over 20 years' experience, I learned a few new tricks myself!

In this book, you will learn about how babies' sleep changes over time, that sleeping like a baby is not what one might think, about how simple things like full tummies and swaddling can be game changers, and how freeing a routine can actually be.

This book is not about 'sleep training'. Instead, it is about empowering parents to understand their babies' sleep patterns. Its power lies in its simplicity. If you are that parent who is getting ready for baby and reading in advance, you will feel well informed about sleep ahead of baby's arrival. If you are an exhausted parent of a 6-month-old, you can pick it up and read the parts that apply to your baby's developmental stage. If you have read a whole chapter but are too tired to remember it (or you are too tired to read a whole chapter), there are crib notes! If you simply cannot believe that these straightforward tips will work in real life, there are real-life examples. If you cannot find your way around a problem, there are troubleshooting tips.

Many parents feel alone. They feel alone with their new baby, alone in the middle of the night, and alone with their new sleepless baby in the middle of the night! Cat and Sarah will make you feel less alone. They will jolly you along. They will help you realise that all those people who had 'perfect babies that slept through from two weeks' were either fibbing or forgetting. They will have your back, from sunup to sundown, and the dark hours in between. And they will help you to get through the first year and beyond with less worry and trepidation. Because most of the time, when you ask yourself 'Is this normal?' they will quietly reassure you that it is.

The Sleep Mums understand that in order to figure out 'how to' parents need to be empowered with the 'why'. Why does my baby wake up so often? Why can't my baby settle? Why is my baby crying?

When parents know 'why', 'how' follows more easily. Cat and Sarah dispense their wisdom with kindness and compassion. They have seen it all when it comes to baby sleep. They know the 'whys'. They will guide you, but they will not judge you.

And that is what this book is. A guide. A North Star for parents to glance up at in the dark of night. A compass to steer them through tricky developmental shifts. A sleep map. A gift.

Enjoy it. Enjoy your baby. And sweet dreams!

Dr Niamh Lynch, Consultant Paediatrician

IG @dr_niamh_lynch
twitter @niamh_dr
Tik Tok @tiktokkiddydoc

Who Are We?

We are The Sleep Mums, Cat and Sarah. We are experts, and we know a lot about baby sleep. We're also parents, so we know how you feel. Exhausted.

We launched our award-winning parenting podcast to support parents with zero-judgement, practical baby sleep advice – advice you can use to help your baby sleep better *and* not make you feel crap about yourself, which so many parenting books tend to do. (They have a habit of tucking guilt inside the covers by implying if you 'do this' or you 'don't do that', you are not doing it correctly.)

So, we want to tell you: you are already doing a great job. Even sleep deprived . . . and we can help you with that, too!

Sarah is a baby-and-child sleep expert, who has been supporting parents to get a good night's sleep for over 20 years. And I'm Cat (the one who got the job to introduce us to you). I'm a broadcaster, journalist and self-confessed parenting-advice junkie. But I definitely don't think there is just one way to parent (Mamakarma would only come and bite me on the bum if I did). Together, we are the Batman and Robin of baby sleep; except we mostly – apart from that one crazy night out – wear our knickers *under* our trousers.

It's lovely to meet you.

Who Are You?

You are a loving parent or caregiver. You would do *anything* to get a good night's sleep.

You might be getting prepared and reading this before baby arrives or as they snooze beside you in those early newborn days, knowing that forewarned is forearmed. Or your eye bags may tell your own bedtime story: you haven't slept in weeks or months.

If your baby is not sleeping, you have not done anything wrong. Your baby is not broken (although *you* might *feel* broken from lack of sleep), and you are not a bad parent. Baby sleep is not linear; it changes a lot during their first few years. They like to keep us on our toes that way. You are here because you want honest support and you need real solutions.

And the good news?

We can give that to you.

This book will arm you with the confidence and tools to see you through the long nights of your baby's wee years.

How to Use This Book

We know you're tired. We know you don't want to read judgemental, outdated and wordy parenting advice that makes you feel like you've failed before you've even started. We will never dictate that you need to be a particular type of person or parent for the guidelines to work. You are you (and we love you for it).

We've split the book into four parts to help you work out where you need to be.

In 'Part I: The Basics', following the introductions, we give you the foundations for our Golden Guidelines. There's the science bit, the disrupting-the-clichés bit – such as 'Why doesn't my baby sleep like one?' – and there's your tool kit. Everything you need to get started.

In 'Part II: The Golden Guidelines', we share the essentials that will help you and your baby towards better sleep. You can dip in and out of them or read them from start to finish. They are roughly chronological, but you may find you need to go back and forth between them, as your needs – like your baby's sleep – will not fall in a straight line. They are designed to be really practical; even just reading the Contents page will give you a starting point for better sleep.

At the beginning of each guideline you will find our Crib Notes. These are your cheat sheets for each chapter, summarising what we want you to take away from it and the key points that will see you through.

As you get stuck into each chapter, we'll explain the rationale behind it and give you the tools you need to make it work for you and your baby, whatever their age. Each guideline ends with a way for you to use it, whether you're in survival mode or you are ready to put it into action and move forwards.

After our guidelines, you will find Part III: 'The Sleep Mums' Routines'. These outline exactly what you are aiming to fit into a day for your baby and a structure for what that could look like. You will also learn how to hack the routines, so that they work for you, and there are examples to give you an idea of how to do it all yourself. (There are also pages at the back of the book where you can write your own routines, if you need to.)

'Part IV: What Do I Do When . . .?' includes our troubleshooting section with real-life questions from parents like you and our answers. It is so important to us to put our advice into practice in the real world, as we do in our podcasts. We are often told that this really helps our listeners – and our readers – to feel less alone.

And finally, there is the 'Break-in-Emergency' chapter – the one to read when it's the middle of the night and you feel like you're the only person in the world who's up and you can't face another day like that. It's there for you whenever you need it.

As are we.

Part I
The Basics

Introduction

We have read a lot of parenting books. One of the things we bonded over in the early days of our friendship was our frustration that the advice in these books always seemed so extreme; if you're 'this' kind of parent or 'that', then you should co-sleep/ make your baby cry it out/do the funky-chicken dance . . . And then your baby will absolutely, positively sleep. But we know from experience of working with thousands of families that that isn't how it works.

It might seem odd at the beginning of a parenting sleep book to tell you that sleep books don't work, but many of them don't. All too often, they fail to equip parents with the confidence, tools and balanced support they need to help their baby to sleep. They tend to be complicated and don't take into account that as well as every child being different, every family is different, too.

Most parents don't want extremes. They usually fall somewhere in the middle, cherry-picking advice from either end of the 'you-must-do-this-to-make-your-baby-sleep' debate. They just want to do what works. For them.

Claire's baby might have been sleeping through at three weeks old when all she did was put him in his crib, sing 'I like Big Butts and I Cannot Lie' and he slept for 12 hours straight. But her hip-hop-loving baby is not your baby, and you are not his parent. Thank goodness. Your little dreamboat is all yours (and, frankly, gorgeous, by the way).

So, if this sleep book isn't like any other parenting sleep book, what is it?

Our Golden Guidelines of baby sleep will give you the knowledge, skills and confidence to help your baby sleep, not just for the next few nights but over the next year and beyond.

After they are born, a baby's mind grows almost as exponentially as your laundry pile. We help and encourage our babies to reach all those wonderful milestones as they learn to sit up, crawl and say their first words. And yet, few parents think of sleep as another milestone that they can help their children towards. Of course, it *can* happen all by itself (like it did for Claire), but there are things we can do as parents and caregivers to create the right environment for better sleep to be established. Just as practising tummy time helps a baby learn how to crawl.

Some children will sleep better than others. But sleep is one of the most important things you can help your baby to do – because they need it to continue their development into adults. And the adults looking after them need sleep, too, to cope with the daily demands of those tiny growing ~~dictators~~ humans!

We want to help you and your family to get more sleep. And our goal is to empower you – to give you practical advice that actually works. Not every one of our Golden Guidelines has to be for you: most will work like a dream, some will take practice and there may be a few that simply do not fit you, your lifestyle or your family.

We will not promise that by reading this you will miraculously get 12 hours each and every night; sleep just doesn't work like that – for anyone. But this is a realistic and supportive guide that will give you an understanding of baby sleep, help you get more of it and be by your side when you feel like it's all gone tits up.

Expectations

Crib Notes

- **Sleeping 'through' means different things to different people.**

- **Night waking is totally normal.**

- **Babies can take time to sleep solidly without wakefulness, requiring settling from you or themselves.**

- **Average night and day sleep varies, depending on age and baby.**

- **Your baby *is* good – however they are sleeping.**

There's a lot of pressure from those around us – and ourselves – when it comes to baby sleep. 'Sleeping through' is such a misleading phrase, because, technically, none of us does. Plus, a good night's sleep means different things to different people. Right now, even 45 minutes might sound good to you; or perhaps you won't accept anything less than a full 8 hours.

That partly explains how a parent's experience of baby sleep can vary so much – not because it actually does, but because of how they interpret it – and why so many of the mums and dads we speak to feel like they are the only ones who have a baby that doesn't sleep.

Also, people fib about baby sleep all the time; whether because they love the drama of it and exaggerate ('You'll never sleep once the baby is here') or because they feel they have to – all parents will have felt the panic when someone asks them if their baby is 'good', when what they are really asking is, 'How do they sleep?' Even if you are so tired you can barely find the words, there is only one answer you feel you should give, 'Yes, of course, they're good'.

So, what is the truth about baby sleep? Baby sleep is different from adult sleep, so our expectations of it should be different, too. Babies do not go from not sleeping through the night to sleeping from 7am to 7pm for ever and ever, happily ever after. It can take around six months for babies, sleep cycles to lengthen and become more similar to an adult's, with lots of changes over the first year and beyond.

And, honestly, sometimes baby sleep can be baffling. You can do all the things you're 'supposed to do' and still have a bad night's sleep. However, we believe that understanding it as far as possible will give you the tools to help you through – if not every night, then most. We will go into more detail about the science of it all in the next chapter.

Understanding Baby Sleep

Crib Notes

- **Your baby is not broken if they are not sleeping well.**

- **Babies don't sleep like adults.**

- **Babies are lighter sleepers.**

- **Baby sleep cycles are usually between 40 and 50 minutes.**

- **Baby sleep cycles begin to lengthen from 6 months.**

Nothing can really prepare you for the tiredness of parenthood. No two nights are the same, and when you get three hours of sleep it feels like you've slept for a fairy-tale hundred years. You think, I've cracked this baby sleep thing; it will only get better from here.

Except you're up the next night. And the next. You're doing the baby dance – the one you used to do in clubs but now do in milk-stained pyjamas because it might, just possibly, help your baby to sleep. 'Help!' you cry, as you shimmy. 'What am I doing wrong?'

We want to make something clear; *you are not doing anything wrong*. You are just learning to be a parent and your little one is learning to be a human. However, there are things we can do as parents and caregivers that help (more than the shimmying), so you both get more sleep.

Sleeping Like a Baby

This well-worn phrase means something very different to how babies actually sleep and has confused generations of parents. So, how do they sleep?

Well, let's start with how *you* sleep. Most adults have a sleep cycle that lasts around 100 minutes. During that time, we go through various stages of sleep, ranging from light to active to quiet and, finally, deep. At the end of a sleep cycle, an adult turns over and goes back to sleep (the mental equivalent of pushing the snooze button) or they wake up. Then actually press the snooze button.

What about babies? Babies haven't mastered the snooze button yet. They're not born with the sleep cycles we take for granted. They are much lighter sleepers than adults but need sleep more than we do. It's crucial for their physical and mental development, helping to establish connections in the brain, which, in turn, helps with language, reasoning and relationships.

Babies' shorter and more active sleep cycles, along with immature nasal passages, mean they can be really noisy when they sleep. It also means they can disturb those sleeping close to them, even when they are finally asleep.

Baby Sleep Cycles

A baby only has two types of sleep (active and quiet), compared to an adult's full range. Their sleep cycles are also shorter, at around 40–50 minutes. It can take up to 6 months for these to lengthen and become more like an adult's. So while baby may sleep 'through' from before 6 months, it can take time for them to do so solidly, without requiring settling from you or by themselves.

Understanding your baby's sleep cycle matters for a number of reasons:

Babies spend more time in active sleep. In active sleep (often called REM), they move their arms and legs more and breathe less deeply. This active, lighter phase of sleep, usually at the start, is one of the big reasons it's really important that they feel comfortable falling asleep where they are going to stay, usually in their cot or crib (as opposed to in your arms).

During this active phase, they may sleep with their eyes not fully closed or even with one eye open, as though they are checking you've not gone to the bathroom on your own (folks, that ship has sailed!). They may also open their eyes fully and have a grunt or a grumble before going back to sleep. Disturbing them in this phase can wake them up, making it harder for them to go back to sleep and complete their snooze cycle.

In the quiet phase of sleep (often called NREM), a baby's breathing deepens and they move less, which can feel scary for new parents. After spending time trying to get them to sleep, ensuring they have passed through the active phase, you can suddenly find yourself desperate to wake them up to make sure they are ok.

If you are ever anxious or concerned, please know that you can check they're ok. You can (usually) do so without waking them: take a few minutes and have a listen; if you are still worried, put a gentle hand on baby or lightly under their nose to feel the warmth of their breath.

If they are older and you are not in the same room as them, we recommend leaving the door ajar, when possible, to make entering and exiting that little bit easier. And quieter.

They will sleep more soundly in this phase, so the arms-to-bed transfer does sometimes work, but we still don't recommend it because the change of environment can be disorientating for baby. We'll go into more detail about how to put your baby to sleep so they are comfortable and aware of where they are under 'Always Put Your Baby to Bed Aware' (see p. 94).

Understanding your baby's sleep cycle helps because it means that if they always wake 40 minutes after you put them down, you know that they are likely to be trying to move between sleep cycles, rather than waking for food.

SURVIVAL:

Daylight is your friend. Use light (real and artificial) to improve baby's circadian rhythm (see Glossary, p. 301). During the day: if in doubt, go out.

MOVING FORWARDS:

Babies can be restless sleepers and do all sorts of weird and wonderful things to try to soothe themselves. If they wake, noisily (and this can include crying) or are moving around a lot, they may just be going between sleep cycles, so give them a chance to settle themselves.

No Rules for Feelings

We take a light-hearted approach to discussing baby sleep, both in our podcast and in writing this book, because often, when parenting, if you don't laugh, you might cry. Then the baby will cry, and before you know it, everyone's crying. So, we joke, but it feels important to say that having a baby can be the punchline to a very hard, long and not-particularly-funny stand-up (or lie-down) routine.

Birth

For many parents, having a newborn might not be the euphoric, life-affirming event they anticipated. It's bloody and messy, and it can feel totally isolating, even though you now have someone with you at all times of day and night. Never alone, but lonely.

You may have had a traumatic birth. Sometimes labours and deliveries are difficult, and there can be conflict with medical professionals over how things play out. Emotionally, it's a lot to cope with and can make the post-natal period feel confusing and unpleasant. You may also feel like this when you've had a technically 'easy' birth, too.

The person who has given birth can feel like a shadow of their old self – deflated, not just in body, but emotionally, too. Like they have been literally ripped in two. Caring for the baby feels like clockwork. One eye always on the time, knowing that they need to feed and change and clothe and burp. So they do it. Or a part of them does.

And partners can feel pretty confused, too. Traumatised by seeing the person they love go through a difficult and sometimes scarily urgent medical experience, where they felt useless. Then, on top of this, they don't always feel they can talk about it or share it because they know their partner is going through the same, and then some.

That's a lot of emotions going on.

Baby Blues

This is not a colour scheme for a nursery. The baby blues supposedly occurs in the week or two after birth and are often explained away by science through hormonal and chemical changes after birth. But for many it lasts longer than that and, frankly, 'the baby blues' sounds flippant in comparison to how it feels.

You may be teary, anxious and feel very up and down. And while the baby-blues cloud will generally lift, with rest, recuperation and some self-love, it's not always as straightforward as it's made to sound.

Post-natal Anxiety (PNA)

Post-natal anxiety usually occurs in the first year after having a baby. It's common to feel some anxiety after you have a baby, for all the reasons mentioned above, but PNA is more than that. It's a feeling of anxiousness that will not go away, and while it can be connected to specific situations, it's more likely to be an overarching feeling. If you are someone who has experienced anxiety before having a baby, it can be more likely to affect you afterwards.

There are a range of different symptoms, including but not restricted to: overwhelming feelings of fear or worry, a racing heart, being unable to sleep (this is important for us to mention because sometimes baby is sleeping fine but you are not, as was the case for Cat after her son was born), a constant worry that something bad is going to happen.

These can all feel really scary. If you think you might be experiencing PNA, please talk to a healthcare professional. Do not feel you need to deal with this alone.

Post-natal Depression (PND)

Post-natal depression is often described by medical professionals as 'feeling down' or a negative mood that lasts for more than two weeks. There is also a lot of confusion and crossover between what people think of as the baby blues, post-natal anxiety and post-natal depression. PND is often used as a kind of umbrella term for all the negative feelings people have after having a baby.

PND symptoms can be similar to those of PNA, including struggling to sleep. You might also lose interest in normal activities, feel hopeless and find it hard to concentrate or eat.

Getting Help

Many new parents (fathers and partners, too) feel sad for lots of reasons, and while we say it's ok to feel those things, it's also important to talk to someone about them. Your mental health is completely separate from the love you feel for your baby. There is no shame in feeling sad or low and not into this parenting gig.

There are varying degrees of all these post-natal feelings and for some people it doesn't always happen in the first few weeks. There are many points in the first year and beyond (up to three years after birth) where you may feel a hormonal imbalance that causes complex emotions and feelings of inadequacy, anxiety and depression. But support is out there, so look for help as soon as possible (see Resources, p. 305).

Sleep is important and we're passionate about helping parents to sleep more. We also know that there's a lot of pressure around sleep, and when these emotions are weighing heavily on you, they can feel heavier than the bundle in your arms. We are here to help and guide you and make you feel supported, but please don't feel like a failure if bits of this book do not work for you.

The Partner Rules

Crib Notes

- Know the guidelines.

- Sign up to Team Baby.

- Be the support they don't need to ask for.

- Listen to them without judgement.

- Learn how your baby likes to be settled (see p. 98).

Whether a new baby makes a family of two, three, four or more, it's always life-changing. And sometimes, one of the hardest things about the first few months is that it's not the same experience for everyone. This can make it so isolating. Even within a couple.

Partners can feel overwhelmed, sometimes a little clueless, and that, in turn, can make them feel helpless. They can also experience post-natal depression and/or anxiety, too. If you're not in a couple, the support of family or friends is important. People talk about a village, but it doesn't need to be. Just being held up by one or two villagers can stop parenthood feeling so big, when your baby is so small.

Rule 1. Team Baby

When it comes to sleep, a united front between parents and caregivers is vital. This is, perhaps, the foremost Partner Rule. You need to agree on how you will help your baby to sleep, what sleep associations and bedtime routine you will use, how you will settle them, what time they will go to bed and when they should get up. And stick to it. Consistency is key for everyone on Team Baby.

It is crucial that one caregiver doesn't decide they want to always swing baby to sleep when the other is going to be up for the rest of the night dealing with the fallout. Decide together and make a plan. It's ok to have slightly different routines: one of our listeners sings her daughter songs, but her dad sounds like his tonsils have been put in a blender when he sings 'Twinkle Twinkle', so he reads a bedtime story instead! But the big decisions need to be made together; and, ideally, not in the middle of the night.

Rule 2. Be as Supportive as a Maternity Bra

Living with a baby is a brave, new, and sometimes scary world. Telling your partner that they're doing a good job, you're proud of them and they're a good parent does more than just soothe a hormonal mind – it makes you and them feel part of a team. They might not feel like they have 'this', but they have you.

But don't try to solve their problems. Listen to them without judgement. Especially when they are full of hor-moans (see Glossary, p. 301). If you are a practical person, you might think that their worries can be solved with a cuppa and some advice.

Don't try to fix things. Sometimes a cry is good. And there may be a lot of tears. That's what those 56 muslins they said you'd need are for.

Encourage them to look for support from groups, even if it seems like they are coping. You cannot be their everything. Finding like-minded parent friends is good for them, and it's good for you, too.

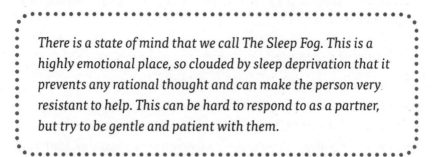

There is a state of mind that we call The Sleep Fog. This is a highly emotional place, so clouded by sleep deprivation that it prevents any rational thought and can make the person very resistant to help. This can be hard to respond to as a partner, but try to be gentle and patient with them.

Rule 3. And Put Your Practical Pants On

Learn how to do the practical baby stuff – bath time, changing nappies and so on. These things are not all just their job, even if they find it hard to let baby go.

An easy way to give some practical support is to take your baby out for a walk in the early evening before bedtime. This will give them a break to wash, have a bath or just gather their strength before the night shift.

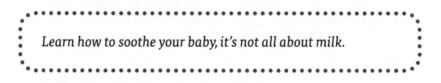

Learn how to soothe your baby, it's not all about milk.

A baby takes up an extraordinary amount of time for a being so small, and there's no luxury of a tea break. So don't make them feel like they are looking after the baby *and* you. And don't wait to be asked; if you see something that needs doing, just do it. If the house is messy, don't give them grief about it – do something about it.

And always get them a drink of water or juice and a snack if they're feeding!

Rule 4. Get Involved

If they want you to, take over one of the night feeds. It doesn't have to be every night, but it's a good way to bond with baby if they feel ready. But don't push them if they're not.

If you're trying to settle baby, tag team as this can be a really emotional and intense thing to do. Sometimes you might need to take the lion's share, even if you're working the next day. It's likely to only be a few days and teamwork can be vital to make this a success, especially when weaning from night feeds.

And last but not least: wind, wind, wind. Whether breast- or bottle-fed, passing baby over after a feed can be a really good way of sharing the bond . . . and the spit up!

Supporting each other is hard but essential. You will argue and bicker but try not to do so in hushed tones over your sleeping baby (which is easily done). Agree on how you can split the load, so both of you know you will get a break at some point.

Your Sleep Tool Kit

'They don't come with a manual.' If you are a parent of a small child or baby, it's likely you've heard this more than once. Personally, we're not sure we would have taken too kindly to being handed one at the same time that our babies were slid wetly on to our chests. But the reason there's no manual is because there's no one right way. Babies might all look like wee old men, but they are, thankfully, all different – and we, as parents, are different, too.

Still, manual or no manual, you can feel unprepared, and wish there was someone to tell you what to do (and preferably not Google at 3am). So, in place of one, we have created a parenting tool kit – a Mary Poppins bag of useful things that will help your baby sleep better.

Environment Matters

When babies are born, you don't want to take your eyes off them for a second, even to blink. They say 'sleep when the baby sleeps', which sounds lovely, but they don't realise THAT INVOLVES CLOSING YOUR EYES!

It is impossible to watch baby all the time, no matter how much you might want to, and an important part of keeping them safe is ensuring that their parents are getting some sleep. So, making a sleeping environment that's as safe as possible is key for baby but is also vital to helping you rest easy.

Back to Sleep

Older generations will often say (unhelpful) things like, 'But we put you to sleep on your tummy/in the footwell of the car/in the street/upside down – and you turned out fine'. But if you follow that logic, we would all still be peeing in sheds in the garden or putting our kids to sleep in the bottom drawer of the night stand.

The Back to Sleep campaign was introduced in the 1990s, and since then, rates of sudden infant death syndrome (SIDS) have dropped by 81 per cent in the UK.* When a baby falls asleep on their tummy, they sleep more deeply, and it can make it hard for them to wake up if their breathing gets interrupted. So, the safest way to put healthy babies to sleep is on their backs until they are at least a year. Once they start rolling over (around 4–6 months), they might move from this position, but still aim to put them down on their backs at the start of any sleep (unless advised differently by a healthcare professional).

Safety Covered

Make sure there's nothing in the sleep space that can cover your baby's head or face while they are sleeping. This includes cot bumpers and lots of cuddly toys. Ideally, use a swaddle in the early days (see p. 26), and any (thin) blankets should be tucked in securely. After they have transitioned from a swaddle, using a baby sleeping bag/sack helps to keep covers and fuss to a minimum, but make sure to use the right size for your baby, so it cannot creep up above their chin.

Put baby down in their cot, so their feet are close to the bottom, giving them lots of clear space for their head and face at the top. Once they are around 6 months and can pull things away from

---

* https://www.lullabytrust.org.uk/ons-2015/

their face, you can consider using a comforter. However, we recommend keeping it to just one toy or blanket (and make sure it is a breathable one) in their cot while sleeping.

Crib Party

It's important to make sure your cot meets the current safety standards, especially if you're buying second-hand (remembering always to buy a new mattress) and that it is built correctly.

Use a firm, well-fitting mattress. Softer isn't safer when it comes to baby, even though it might seem a bit medieval to put them on such a firm mattress. A solid sleep space is crucial for their physical development and much safer than a soft one, which might dip at the edges and allow them to get stuck down the sides.

Another thing you need to think about in terms of baby's cot is where to put it. Be mindful of drafts and secure any nearby pictures and cords or wires from a monitor. Think about the position of the cot in terms of when baby is on the move and ensure that there's nothing close by that they could use to climb out.

Close Sleeping

The NHS guidelines say that baby should sleep in your room for the first six months. These are only guidelines, though, and it will often depend a little on your own personal set-up. Some babies will need to stay in your room much longer than six months and for others this may be impractical – for example, if you or a partner (or another child) are disturbing baby, that's not going to help anyone get a good night's sleep. We all have different homes with different set-ups and parents need to consider how they feel about having baby in the room with them and for how long, and what will work best for their family.

There are a few reasons why sharing a room with your baby can be beneficial, some of which are biological. When you safely sleep with or very close to your baby it is like there is an invisible string connecting you. Incredibly, you help to regulate some of your baby's physiological responses – like heart rate, brain waves, sleep states, oxygen levels, temperature and breathing. Which means that if anything stops working as well as it should, that connection can act like a pull-in-emergency cord.

Some parents also choose to share a bed with their baby (known as co-sleeping). If this is what you would like to do, you need to know how to do it safely. Please check out the Lullaby Trust for best practice (see Resources, p. 305).

Can I Take Your Temperature?

Keeping baby's sleeping environment at the same temperature as much as possible is important, the optimum temperature being between 16 and 20°C.

Put them in a single layer, like a sleepsuit (include a vest if they're small or if it's cold), then put them in a swaddle or baby sleeping bag, depending on their age. If needed, use thin, breathable blankets and layer them, if required.

Sssssh . . . it

For a baby, whose senses are just beginning to explode, bright lights, sounds, music, TVs, mobile phones – pretty much all the trappings of modern life – can make the world feel like a nightclub. It's been a long time since we set foot in a club, but even so, you don't normally sleep in one. To combat all these variables, there are tools we can use to make their sleep environment a more consistent space. One of these is sound.

Strangely, a random noise like a dog barking, a car alarm, that third creaky floorboard from the right can all easily wake your baby, whereas a constant sound that they can tune into can keep other noises from disturbing them.

Using a sound that you are in control of – like white noise (see p. 25) – can give you the confidence to behave in your home as you would normally and avoid literally tiptoeing around them.

Here are a few things to think about:

- You will be listening to the white noise for a long time, so choose something you can tolerate.
- We recommend using it from birth . . .
- . . . but you don't have to!
- Turn off for feeds, so it doesn't lull baby to sleep during feeding.
- If you introduce a noise weeks or months after birth, one that you have naturally been making will work better – for example, if you always shush when your baby goes to sleep, go for a shushing sound.
- Once you have decided which noise you are going to use, be consistent with your choice (see Be Consistently Consistent, p. 71); it can take time for baby (and you) to get used to it, so if you feel it's not working right away, don't just stop using it.
- Use your noise for all naps and overnight. Initially, play it for the duration of any sleep and if you are out and about, always take it with you.
- Make it easy for yourself – it needs to be accessible and portable.

When thinking about the volume of the noise you choose, you want it to be somewhere around the noise of a dishwasher and louder than you think (roughly 50–60 decibels).

To wean baby off their noise when you feel the time is right, start with the volume higher when they are settling, then reduce it once they are settled. Only increase it again for settling. Over the course of a few weeks, you can reduce the volume completely, until it is off during deeper sleep and just becomes a settling tool. There is no hurry to stop using a sleep sound, though.

The longer-term aim can be to use it to trigger sleep, but this only comes with repetition and often doesn't happen until between 12 and 18 months.

White Noise

It's likely that before you became a parent you hadn't heard much about white noise but in the baby charts, this guy is bigger than The Beatles. White noise is a blend of all audible sound frequencies. It produces a 'shush' sound, similar to what your baby heard in the womb. By balancing out all other sounds, it allows babies (and adults) to switch off and get to sleep. It also works to keep the sound environment consistent and controlled by you.

Never worry about normal household sounds – flush the toilet, put on the washing machine and watch TV. Your baby isn't used to quiet, so you don't need to sit in silence (although you may want to!).

You do not need to buy a white-noise gadget – there are plenty of videos online and apps. Use white noise for as long as you or baby/child wants.

Pink Noise

Where white noise cancels out other sounds, pink noise – things like rainfall, leaves rustling or whale sounds – is meant to make us feel calmer. It works in much the same way as white noise but on slightly different sound frequencies.

These more ambient sounds can be more disturbing, depending on the person; some people love to listen to waves crashing on a beach, but for others it just really makes them need a wee!

We recommend white noise (over pink noise); not because it's a magic trick that will instantly settle your baby, but it is the glue gun of your tool kit – something that can hold it all together by aiding deeper and less-disrupted sleep.

Sleep Supporters

We are your biggest sleep supporters when it comes to helping your baby to sleep better. However, as well as us, we'd like to introduce you to a couple of other excellent sleep supporters. In the guidelines, you will find these referred to as sleep associations and comforters, but here are our top two:

Every Day I'm Swaddling

Swaddling, if done safely, is like a lullaby in material form. Formed from a large muslin or a breathable blanket, a swaddle can soothe baby to sleep, make them feel safe, keep them calm, cosy and, importantly, more likely to sleep soundly. It is most helpful during the first few months of baby's life as it replicates the feeling of being inside (. . . as in, the womb, not jail!).

The science bit is that swaddling can help baby to not be disturbed by their own startle (or Moro) reflex (see Glossary, p. 301), which can jolt them awake when they least expect (and you least want) it.

Swaddling looks like origami when you first get started and it can be hard to work it out. Babies often fight the swaddle, too, leaving parents to presume that they don't like it. It is worth persevering with, though, as in many ways it acts as baby's first comforter.

Swaddling, Step by Step

Step 1

Fold your swaddle square into a large triangle. When your baby is tiny you want the triangle to meet itself at the bottom. This makes it safer because you have less excess material at the bottom and, as your baby grows, you can simply move the triangle up.

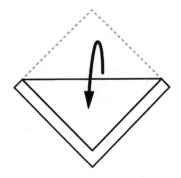

Step 2

Place your baby so their feet are pointing towards the point of the triangle and shoulders are in line with the straight edge. Flatten and stretch the swaddle underneath.

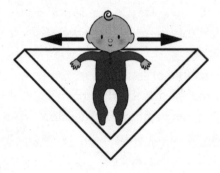

Step 3

Take one edge of the swaddle and stretch it over their chest. Wrap it snuggly underneath your baby, keeping the opposite arm on top. To get a snug fit, roll baby onto their side, allowing you to get the swaddling blanket right under their back.

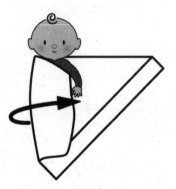

Step 4

Take the opposite edge and wrap it over your baby, folding in their free arm and coming right across and fully under them.

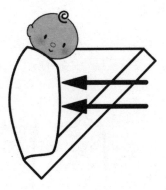

Step 5

When swaddling your baby, make sure their arms are comfortably by their sides or coming across to meet at their tummy. This little bit of pressure on the tummy can help comfort and release any wind.

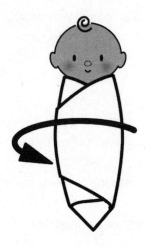

Step 6

Once baby is snug as a bug, gently hold their knees and push the legs into the froggy position to check for free hip movement. The swaddle should be secure across their chest and looser around the hips and legs.

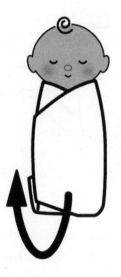

Transitioning out of a swaddle

There isn't a specific age when you should stop swaddling, but once baby can roll over or push themselves up, it's no longer safe for them to be swaddled.

Signs that your baby might be ready to break out of the swaddle:

- Increasing noise from them overnight as they fight with the swaddle
- Unsettled naps and overnight sleep, having been previously settled
- Starting to show signs of rolling over

Step 1

Start by slightly loosening the fabric across the second arm, ensuring it is still snug enough that it will not become loose, but loose enough that baby can start to wriggle their arm a bit more. Do this for approximately three nights.

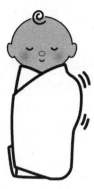

Step 2

Once your baby has become used to the increased arm movement, swaddle with the second arm on top. The other arm is still swaddled snugly and the chest is secure, but one arm is completely loose. Do this for three nights, or longer if baby is now comfortable with this transition.

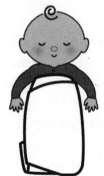

Step 3

Next, swaddle around baby's chest with both arms out.

You are now ready to transition to a sleeping bag.

Note: swaddling is not considered safe if you are co-sleeping.

Comfort Sleeping

Comforters are like an extension of you – something that can consistently give your baby comfort. They can be almost anything, and even if not initially chosen by you, they are reinforced by you, so you do have control over them. Sarah has a client whose kid chose their dad's (clean) boxers; the parents were happy enough and at least they wash easily!

We often recommend muslins as comforters, as your baby will have seen one on you at almost all times. They smell like home (and maybe a little milky), and they are easily replaced, washed and repurposed. Plus, bigger kids can take a wee square of their muslin tucked in their pocket when they head off to school.

Comforters can be introduced to your baby's sleeping area from 6 months. It can be a good idea for you to sleep with or carry one against your body the day or night before introducing one to make it smell like you.

Soothers or dummies fall into the category of comforters, too, as do fingers and thumbs – yours and theirs. Just remember, though, you can't leave your finger with them all the time (it makes spreading toast very difficult)!

It's a Gas

We're like a 5-year-old with fart gags when it comes to winding – we talk about it all the time! The reason it matters is it really can be the difference between a good feed/nap/day sleep/night sleep/alllll the sleep . . .

Baby wind is usually caused by air that your little one has taken in during feeding, crying and yawning. If they don't get rid of it, it can become very painful. By about the age of 6 months, most babies are moving around more and, like adults, are more able to dispel their own wind. However, we recommend you continue to wind them for their first year.

Common signs of wind are squirmy, unsettled periods, arching back, outbursts of painful crying and uncomfortable expressions when they are lying flat or being held upright.

On p. 56, we share all the ways to help wind your baby, with illustrations, and you should find there the one that works best for you and them. The most important thing about having these techniques in your tool kit, though, is to remember to use them every single time you feed. There will be times when baby will not bring up a burp, but that doesn't mean they will never need your help getting it out.

Winding can also become a comforting part of your routine. The cuddle-close position you can have your baby in, the rubbing and patting are lovely things for you and baby to share, so even when they no longer need help to dislodge it, you may find you want to keep doing it.

Winding, Step by Step (see p. 56 for illustrations)

- Lift your baby up to your shoulder. Making sure you always support the head and neck, switch between patting and rubbing the whole back. Ensure you have your baby in a hold, which means if they jump or squirm you are supporting them.
- Sit baby on your knee with one hand supporting their neck and back (thumb and fingers below their armpits and one or two fingers supporting their head) and the other hand on

their front, around their chest. Gently rock them back and forth to try to dislodge any air bubbles.

- Have your baby sitting on your knee with a nice straight back; support their front and back and move them in circular motions.
- Lie your baby on their tummy across your knees, supporting their neck, and rub their back in big motions all over.
- Use your whole hand (thumb on one side and fingers on the other) on baby's back to massage/gently compress up the whole length of their sides, either side of their spine. If baby squirms, rub or pat here as there is likely a bit of trapped wind. We call this one 'Incy Windy Spider', as the motion is a little like a spider crawl up either side.
- When baby is out of the newborn stage, you can also lie them on their back and gently cycle their legs. This puts a little pressure on their lower intestine and can help push out a parp!

Use all the techniques in your parenting bag to wind your baby.

Super Settling

Settling techniques are one of the most important tools to have in your parenting back pocket. (Well, settling techniques and wipes.) You need these less in the early days as baby is usually settled by things we already need to do – feeding, winding, sucking, swaddling, rocking, cuddling. However, as they grow, their settling requirements will change. We can't tell you exactly what these will be for you and your baby. However, here are some of the things that you may find useful:

- The Sleep Mums' Shoogle (a very gentle rock – see Glossary, p. 301)
- Tummy rubbing
- Hand holding
- Face rubbing
- Bottom patting
- Back rubbing
- Supported tummy with bottom patting

Make a Plan

We love a plan. Tiredness makes you more impulsive and very few good ideas come in the middle of the night when you've been up for 24 hours straight. If you are going to be making any changes to sleep routines or set-ups, write them down, know how you're going to tackle things and try to stick to the plan.

Take notes on your phone or use the pages we've included at the back of the book for you to write in.

The Sleep Mums' 30-minute Buffer

We wanted to find a happy place between creating routines that give structure while meeting your baby's needs and giving you some flexibility. With that in mind, The Sleep Mums' 30-minute Buffer is a half-hour cushion either side of all the timings in our routines. This means you can follow your baby's cues for sleep, feeds and play and not be a slave to a tight schedule. It also gives you some flexibility to work your day around any plans and . . . well, a buffer when you want to try hacking our routines.

Look After Yourself

It's easy to put yourself last when you become a parent. But looking after yourself is one of the most important things you can do for your baby. Drinking water, going to the toilet by yourself or having a shower are needs. They are not self-care, which sounds more like a spa day (and would be lovely, by the way).

When we talk about looking after yourself, 'what you need' will be different for everyone. But even knowing what that is when you're tired can be difficult, so simply asking for help can be a good place to start. Take up offers from friends and family and always know it's ok to tap out for a while if you need to.

PART II
The Golden Guidelines

The No-rules Rule: the First Two Weeks

Crib Notes

- **It's all an adjustment: you are getting to know yourself as a parent, your baby and your new set-up – it takes time.**

- **Focus on feeds rather than sleep.**

- **Its ok to need help.**

- **And it's ok to say no.**

If, during the first few weeks of baby's arrival, you want to cuddle them all day, every day, that is totally and completely fine. If you really don't, and you're all touched out (see p. 92)? Also fine. You want to dress your baby up as a strawberry and post it on social media? Acceptable. Want to close the door and not see anyone in person or online? You go right ahead.

Allow yourself and your immediate family those first few weeks to get to know your baby and for them to get to know you. Nothing that you do in the early weeks will have a long-term detrimental effect on baby's sleep. The only thing you should concentrate on is making sure baby is fed every two to two and a half hours. Apart from that, don't worry about any rules or guidelines. It's a free for all – the Spring Break of parenting.

In the week after birth (usually three or four days after), there can be a lot of hormonal changes for the postpartum parent that feel fairly wild. This is when there is a decrease of pregnancy hormones and an increase of breastfeeding hormones (even when you are not breastfeeding). You may feel pretty overwhelmed. So, cut yourself some slack: rest, recuperate and try to get some sleep.

On the other hand, you might still feel totally high on birth. Floating on a cloud of muslins, giddy on one snifter of your baby's head. But, also, you might not. Like we said, there are no rules.

And babies know there are no rules in the first few weeks, too. Some are intent on making sure the world knows about their arrival. Others can be very sleepy, making you feel like this parenting game is a skoosh.

Once baby gets used to their new living quarters, they can start to 'wake up' more, particularly at night. The reason for this is that during pregnancy they were rocked to sleep during the day by movements and noise and did their growing and exploring at night. Simply put, your baby is jet-lagged and by now you're probably feeling it, too.

If you are feeling keen, there are two things in the first couple of weeks you can think about when it comes to baby sleep.

The first is helping your baby with their jet lag (also known as 'day and night confusion'):

- During the day, when baby is awake and feeding, keep things bright and light. Open windows and, if you want to, go out to get some fresh air.
- Feed your baby every two and a half hours or less during the day, waking them for a feed if they are asleep. You want to ensure baby's longest stretch of sleep is at night.
- Although it's important to differentiate between night and day, you can use their cot as a safe space for them to have a wriggle, while you shower or get dressed.

- At night, feed your baby whenever they wake. If baby is gaining weight and there are no medical issues, aim to try to keep at least two hours between feeds.
- At night, do all feeding, cuddling, nappy changes in dim or dark conditions and avoid singing, chatting or playing, so they know that it is night-time. 'Night' should be a twelve-hour period, starting sometime between 6 and 8pm.
- Swaddle safely for all sleep, unless co-sleeping.
- But remember to unswaddle – and possibly undress your baby – for feeds to make sure they wake up and stay awake while feeding.

The second thing to think about is making sure your baby takes full, satisfying and consistent feeds (See 'Always Give Your Baby Full Feeds', p. 42). Milk feeds and sleep are inseparable; if they could snuggle up and spoon each other, they would. But what exactly is a full feed? Surely some of us are nibblers and others can eat like a bear? Well, yes, appetites vary, but if your baby falls asleep after a few minutes, it's possible that they haven't had enough, so rouse them and offer more, so you can feel confident that they've had enough.

But wait, you're thinking. I thought this was a sleep book? Don't I want my baby to fall asleep?

Well, yes. But if baby hasn't had enough milk they will not sleep for very long, which is often exhausting for everybody. Focus on keeping baby awake during feeds and the sleep bit will come. There are a few ways to keep them focused on the boob or bottle: strip them down to their vest or nappy, so they're not too warm and cosy, rub their hands or feet and make sure you burp them thoroughly (see p. 33).

It is entirely possible that the first two weeks are totally smooth going and then the day that your partner or family member goes back to work it all goes tits up. (And the worst thing is they won't even believe you!) Don't panic, though, take a breath and follow our guidelines.

The Fourth Trimester

Some people call the newborn stage the fourth trimester, as it's a transition phase for you and baby from pregnancy to life outside. The thinking is that baby stays calmer if they become accustomed to the world more gradually, using techniques like ensuring they're wrapped (ideally swaddled, see page 26) safely when asleep, cuddling them, keeping them close, plenty of skin-to-skin time, shushing, white noise, rocking and swaying. Giving lots of opportunities to suck if you're breastfeeding and skin-to-skin when bottle-feeding can also help.

For many people, this phase might not last a full three months; some find that they start to come out of the intense part of this transition around two months after baby arrives. But remember, it's Spring Break – anything goes!

SURVIVAL:
Just do what you need to do; don't worry about anything or anyone else.

MOVING FORWARDS:
Focus on giving baby full feeds and think about when day and night are for you and your family.

Always Give Your Baby Full Feeds

Crib Notes

- Babies need a feed every two to four hours until 6 months.

- Keep baby awake during feeds.

- Baby will not take a full feed without winding.

- Each and every feed counts.

- A full feed can come from breast or bottle.

- Babies differ in how much and how quickly they take what they need for a full feed.

One of the most important things when it comes to sleep is that your baby takes full feeds.

Whether you are breast- or bottle-feeding, you can make sure your baby is getting full and satisfying feeds by following a feeding routine, keeping them awake during feeds, offering them the breast or bottle until you are satisfied that they are full and winding them during and after every single feed.

On Demand

Feeding on demand is where you follow your baby's cues for how often to feed them. In the early days, if you are breastfeeding, feeding on demand can be a great way to develop your feeding relationship with your baby.

However, there are a couple of reasons why feeding on demand might not work for you. If your baby is sleepy, they may not ask for food as regularly as they or you need them to. Also, it can be hard on parents to know what their baby is really asking for: it is not always about milk.

It takes time to get to know your baby. If they are very unsettled and restless, feeding them every time they cry can cause you both difficulties: from a very tired and windy baby to very sore and cracked nipples.

While you are learning your baby's hunger signs, we recommend sticking to the times between day feeds as suggested in our routines. As a guide, this will be between two and four hours, depending on baby's age. Following a routine will help baby to take full feeds. However, that does not mean you cannot feed them in between if they ask for it or you feel you need to feed them. This is all part of you and your baby learning to communicate with each other.

Other exceptions are growth spurts (which happen a lot in the first year, when you may find you need to feed your baby more regularly), when they are teething or simply inconsolable and self-care (sometimes it can be about you, too) – either because you want to or you need to, particularly if you have to relieve pressure if you are breastfeeding.

After the first few weeks, allow baby to sleep until they wake up by themselves at night, unless there is a medical or weight-related reason why they need to be fed more regularly.

> *Always time your baby's feeds from the start of one feed to the start of the next.*

Cluster Feeding

Cluster feeding is when your baby groups several feeding sessions into a short period of time. It's like a rugby team going to an all-you-can-eat buffet. Most newborns will cluster at some point. If it's driven by baby, it tends to happen in the evening when they are tired. This can make it feel like a marathon feeding session and be exhausting for you and them. But cluster feeds can be a good thing because they can mean a fuller tummy. As long as you do what we call 'planned clustering'.

Rather than this chow-down being at the booby or bottle call of your baby, a planned cluster-feeding session can help your baby to sleep longer during the night, which means it can also help you to sleep longer at night, recharging your bones and, if breastfeeding, your milk supply. But how do you plan a cluster?

As you will see in our suggested routines (see part III), we have clustered a couple of feeds together in the late afternoon and early evening. It's also important for you to have a good meal around this time, too, to give you the strength to take on a rugby team!

> *A cleverly planned cluster feed can increase your supply and help baby through any growth spurts that leap up on you.*

Understanding Full Feeds

It can be really hard to know if baby is taking full feeds, so the best thing to look out for is how content they are. If a baby is fully satisfied, then they are likely to sleep better, and if they are well fed and sleep better, they are generally more content.

What is snacking? This is when your baby falls asleep during a feed or becomes unsettled and fussy. This can be interpreted as baby being full, so you move on to the next stage of the routine, but it can mean that they don't take a full feed and quickly become hungry again.

Are Dream Feeds the Dream?

A dream feed is when you gently rouse your baby – usually without fully waking them – to give them a feed before you go to bed. Essentially, you top them up in the hope it will keep them fuller for longer and allow you to get a little more sleep. Occasionally, parents are also advised to do so for medical reasons and/or weight gain.

In the first few weeks of your baby's life you may find yourself offering an unintentional dream feed; if they have been sleeping near you in the evening and you move them when you are ready to go to bed, they often stir, so you give them a feed. It can work well at this early stage but as they grow it often becomes less helpful. They will take the feed and still wake up at the same time they would have done naturally, with or without the dream feed.

You can stop offering a dream feed simply by not doing it and seeing when your baby wakes up. If this seems too daunting, you can reduce the amount you offer for a few nights until you are no longer feeding or by varying the time you rouse your baby for a dream feed. This prevents a habit forming and allows you to see if it impacts the time of their next wake up at all (it usually doesn't).

Giving a full dream feed can be difficult because your baby is sleepy. This means they take less and/or allow more air in (because they are too tired to latch properly) and it can be hard to wind them fully if you are trying to keep them dozy.

The Full-tummy Lowdown

If your baby falls asleep before you have finished feeding them, don't put them down. Wake them up and continue feeding. It feels crazy to wake baby when they look so lovely and peaceful, and you may well feel desperate for a bit of peace and quiet. However, if baby doesn't take a full feed, they will wake up sooner rather than later. Ultimately, letting them fall asleep on the job gets you less sleep, not more.

- Keep your baby awake during feeds by stripping them down to their nappy.
- Rub their hands and feet to keep them on the bottle or boob.
- Try to get to know when your baby is actively sucking and swallowing and when they are using you, or a bottle, as a dummy. Don't feel daft if you don't know early on. As a guideline, if you are feeding more than twice a night by 4–5 months or more than once after 6 months, it is likely that baby is using you or the bottle for comfort rather than hunger. If you are ok with that and you are getting sleep, it

doesn't need to be a problem, but if you're ready to move forwards, you need to find other ways to settle your baby.

- Try to maintain our guidelines of time between feeds. It means your baby will be hungrier and take more at each feed, and they should be less prone to snacking. If your baby only takes small feeds, they will need more of these to fulfil their nutritional needs.

Remember, you and your baby are just working this out together. It's totally normal to not know at the start when baby is full – it's why having a routine can be invaluable. But wouldn't it be so much easier if they just had a gauge to tell you when their tank was full?

If you're wondering whether formula, combination or breastfeeding will help your baby sleep better, there is no straightforward answer. All babies are different. The key when it comes to feeding your baby is that it is personal, and you need to do whatever makes family life work best for you. The human body is amazing, and it blows our minds that we can feed and nourish our babies with it. The human brain is incredible, and it blows our minds that with the right formula, science helps us feed and nourish our babies. Basically, human beings are brilliant.

How to Give Full Feeds

The two of us have breastfed, bottle-fed, combination-fed. Basically, between us we have fed our babies as you would hope any parent would do – however they need to be fed. We are not here to pass judgement – it is about what is best for you and your baby.

There are a few differences, though, in the ways we feed when it comes to giving our babies full feeds.

Breastfeeding

You *can* have a baby that sleeps well and is breastfed. In the early days, breastfeeding babies will nurse often at night. This is firstly because they are encouraging your milk supply, secondly because their stomachs are small and they digest the milk quickly, and thirdly because you produce more prolactin at night – the stuff that makes the white stuff. Your body is kinda like a late-night venue!

Once your milk comes in you will see a change in baby's feeds. They will begin to take bigger feeds and manage to last longer between them. Some babies are quick and will only feed for five to ten minutes on each boob; others can take half an hour on each side. Over time, you will settle into a natural rhythm. The important thing, however your baby feeds, is that they are content until their next one.

Breastfeeding Guide for Full Tummies
- Baby should feed off the first breast and be allowed to come off naturally. Wind baby thoroughly.
- Offer baby the same breast until they again come off naturally. Wind thoroughly.
- Offer baby the first boob a third time to make sure it's fully drained and empty. Wind thoroughly.
- Offer baby the second breast. Wind thoroughly.
- Then offer and wind again.
- Repeat if required.

Not all babies will come off naturally. Look for them stopping the active suck and take them off. You will not know this from the beginning, so just keep watching and looking for clues, which include swallowing, and their jaw and ear lobe moving. Once they stop the active suck for an extended period, it can turn into a comfort suck and go on indefinitely.

This may sound like a lot of offering of breasts. You might even feel like a bit of a boob pusher. However, it means that baby will completely drain the first breast before you offer them the other one. An empty boob means less-blocked ducts, better supply, fuller baby and more sleep.

You should do the above at every single feed. We know it sounds endless, but it is the most efficient way to feed. Some babies will refuse the third or fourth offer. This doesn't mean you should stop offering so many times; it just means that we all have different milk supplies at different times and babies have different levels of hunger at different times.

This works if you're trying to increase your supply because the more you offer, the more your body will create to feed your baby.

It also works if you feel you have an over-supply of milk, as baby will reject it when they are full. As long as you look out for the active suck and swallow.

You should offer like this until you find your own pattern with your baby. Babies tend to become more efficient as they get older.

Bottle-feeding

All babies differ in how much they drink and how quickly they take what they need to be full. However, every baby will wake up to feed at night, whether they are bottle- or breastfed. It's a well-rinsed parenting myth that formula-fed babies sleep better. If you're a sleep-deprived parent who's bottle feeding, you will be glad to know you are not alone.

In fact, research suggests that there is no difference in sleep between formula-fed and breastfed babies. It is true that babies digest formula milk more slowly so they might feed less overall. However, it's important to remember that food isn't the only reason that your baby will wake up. Babies vary in both age and weight when they are able to go through the night without feeding.

There is a huge number of different formulas out there and it is impossible to say which one will be right for your baby. Do not feel you need to stick with the one you started with or the one you used with another child; formulas are always changing. If you feel like it really doesn't suit your baby, switch it up.

The guidelines on the back of formula packets for the amount of milk that baby needs at each age are just that – guidelines. Go with your own baby. As long as they are lasting between feeds, gaining weight, having wet nappies and healthy poos, then they're getting enough. That could be more or less than what it says on the tin and it may vary at different feeds.

Bottle-feeding Guide for Full Tummies
- To get a good full feed, take baby off the bottle every 30–50ml to give yourself time to wind them and them time to digest. You may have heard this called 'pacing'.
- Try to always have milk at a consistent temperature for each feed (refer to your bottles' guidelines on how to warm).
- All bottles are not born the same: some have quirky little air vents that need to be on the top when feeding and close to babies' nose.
- Although there are recommendations for ages on different teats, your baby might not be ready to move on to the faster flow at these times.
- Make sure you know your bottle and teats before you start feeding with a new one.

- After 6 months, if you want to move from a bottle to a beaker-style cup, you can do this as a gradual introduction by choosing one feed a day to swap out.

Combination-feeding

There are many ways to nourish your baby and ensure a full tummy. One that often falls under the radar is combination-feeding, and a number of positive things can come from this, including allowing a partner or another caregiver to be more involved.

Funnily enough, combination-feeding can be done in a combination of ways. It could be breastfeeding and formula-feeding or breastfeeding and giving expressed breast milk in a bottle, or a combo of these.

Some parents start combination-feeding when their baby is a newborn; others breastfeed before switching at some point down the road. And sometimes multiples, maternal health or the health of the baby mean that combination-feeding is a necessity.

If you are breastfeeding and want to combination-feed on the odd night, it can take some pressure off and allow you to recharge your batteries. However, you may need to be aware of your supply or pump to compensate for any missed feeds. You can also choose a feed or feeds to swap out, so your partner, another caregiver – or you – can do it regularly as a bottle-feed. If you do it at the same time every day, it will allow your boobs to get used to it and should not affect your supply for other feeds.

Combination-feeding Guide for Full Tummies
- You can introduce a bottle at any time.
- Try to make sure everyone is calm. If you or baby are not feeling calm, it is better to leave it until another time than to simply persevere.

- To make the transition easier, think about timings, baby's position and environment, keeping these similar to what you've been doing when breastfeeding.

Follow our guide on how to give baby a bottle (see below).

Try to ignore the noise from others who think you should be feeding your baby differently. Many well-meaning folk (like Janet, or perhaps your own mum or mother-in-law) may have surprisingly firm ideas about your boobs or bottles. And it can be so hard to juggle the baby in your arms and all these opposing views. We would love to be there to tell the onlookers that the only best way is the one you have taken. So, feel free to do so on our behalf!

How to Help Baby Take a Bottle
Babies are demanding – and they don't like change. That means introducing a bottle can sometimes be difficult, particularly if your baby is used to being breastfed. And the older they are, sometimes the more resistant they can become.

You've tried. Your partner has tried. Granny has tried. Your baby just won't take a bottle. After a few minutes, you give up and offer the boob. We understand. It's frustrating. But, we promise, your baby will take one. Here are some ways that can help encourage your baby to take a bottle. If not today, that's ok, try again tomorrow. Or the next day. Or the next. Take it one day at a time. You will get there.

- **The warm-up** Baby's milk in a bottle needs to be on the warmer side, as they are used to it being body temperature: not too hot, not too cold.
- **Top teats** Bottles and teats can be very different, from shape to flow for baby, to how they fit in your hand. The right teat shape is one that fits in your baby's mouth without letting any air in. It can be hard to find the one that seals the deal, but it's worth experimenting if your baby is struggling.
- **Pass the bottle** There's a lot going on for you and baby, and it's emotionally and physically different from breastfeeding, so it can be easier to let someone else try. They can wear something of yours or go skin-to-skin to recreate the comfort the baby might be used to.
- **Teat tickle** It can be tempting if it's a struggle to get baby to take the bottle to just try to shove it in and hope for the best. Gently tickling the teat down from their nose or on their cheek means your baby will open their mouth wider and be more ready to accept the bottle.
- **Straight up** Try a straighter feeding position: sitting upright in the crook of your arm or with their back against your tummy. This can help with the flow and stop too much air getting in and causing more wind. Fill the teat with milk to eliminate air, keep the bottle horizontal and tip the bottle up a little, so the milk flows into their mouth more slowly.
- **Bottle hop** Your baby needs to be encouraged to suck the teat by a little milk dropping on to their tongue. One way to do this is for you to do the work for them. Bob, bounce, squat with baby in your arms; this movement helps get the flow started, so they know what they need to do.
- **Suck-cess** Try not to worry if it doesn't happen immediately. If you have a timescale, give yourself time

before the deadline to make it less stressful. Your baby might not feed from the bottle, but they will feed off your anxiety. Take a breath and try another day; success is just around the corner.

> *Once baby is over 5 months, you can go straight to a follow-on beaker, rather than trying with a bottle first.*

SURVIVAL:
Simply focus on giving full feeds and winding.

MOVING FORWARDS:
Try to learn your baby's cues for both hunger and tiredness. Writing it down can help as they can be similar. You will find that if you have a routine, it is likely to help you read your baby better.

Wind Your Baby Longer Than You Think

Crib Notes

- All babies need winding.

- Wind can be one of the biggest disturbances to sleep.

- Baby is unlikely to be able to sleep well until they get their wind out.

- Most babies will need your help to get rid of wind up until 6 months . . .

- . . . but we recommend continuing to wind them after that.

All babies, big and small, bottle- and breastfed, need winding. It is a really important part of feeding and getting a good night's sleep. Even the tiniest air bubble can expand and cause discomfort, especially when a baby is laid down to sleep. It might not happen every time, but they can't tell you when it's brewing. It's better to cover your bases and always wind baby thoroughly. (A surprising amount of parenting falls under 'just in case'.)

If you are bottle-feeding, there will be natural pauses when you can pop baby upright and wind them. Not only does this help prevent trapped wind, it stops baby from gulping their milk too quickly, which can cause wind in itself. If you are breastfeeding, there are also natural pauses when you should wind. When baby comes off the boob themselves, pop them upright and wind them, before returning them to the breast or finishing the feed.

How to Wind

- Lift your baby up to your shoulder. Making sure you always support the head and neck, switch between patting and rubbing the whole back. Ensure you have your baby in a hold, which means if they jump or squirm you are supporting them.

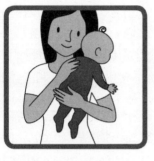

- Sit baby on your knee with one hand supporting their neck and back (thumb and fingers below their armpits and one or two fingers supporting their head) and the other hand on their front, around their chest. Gently rock them back and forth to try to dislodge any air bubbles.

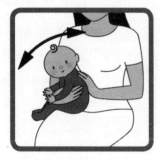

- Have your baby sitting on your knee with a nice straight back; support their front and back and move them in circular motions.

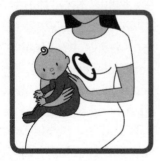

- Lie your baby on their tummy across your knees, supporting their neck, and rub their back in big motions all over.

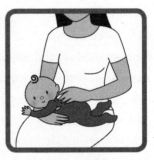

- Use your whole hand (thumb on one side and fingers on the other) on baby's back to massage/gently compress up the whole length of their sides, either side of their spine. If baby squirms, rub or pat here as there is likely a bit of trapped wind. We call this one 'Incy Windy Spider', as the motion is a little like a spider crawling up either side.

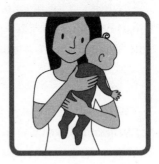

When baby is out of the newborn stage, you can also lie them on their back and gently cycle their legs. This puts a little pressure on their lower intestine and can help push out a parp!

Use all the techniques in your parenting bag to wind your baby.

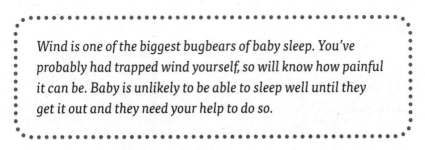

Wind is one of the biggest bugbears of baby sleep. You've probably had trapped wind yourself, so will know how painful it can be. Baby is unlikely to be able to sleep well until they get it out and they need your help to do so.

Wind and Spit-up

Sometimes, when winding your baby, there might be an air bubble trapped behind the milk they have just drunk. This means that when they bring up a burp, they will bring up milk, too. It's often a small amount but can look like a lot and be quite disconcerting. It's one of the (many) reasons everyone tells you you can't have enough muslins.

However, a lot of trapped-wind symptoms can cross over with those of reflux or allergy. If you are concerned, please contact your healthcare professional.

When babies are born their digestive systems haven't fully developed, so they can be more prone to reflux. This is where the contents of their tummy flow back up and sometimes results in spit-up or being sick. It can also make baby more unsettled after a feed, so keeping them upright afterwards can help. It is very common but varies a lot between babies (see Silent Reflux in Glossary, p. 303). If your baby isn't gaining weight and seems to be unhappy a lot of the time, contact your GP.

Winding By Age

0–3 months
- Hold head and neck safely while winding.
- Wind all the time, even when having a cuddle.
- Baby will often bring up milk with a burp.
- Always keep a muslin close.

3 months +

- Use sitting techniques, as described above.
- Always keep a muslin close.
- Babies can spit up more when they are teething.

SURVIVAL:

Try out different winding techniques and find one that works for you and your baby.

MOVING FORWARDS:

Winding baby after a feed means that they will usually wake up a little. This will make it easier for you to work on putting them down in their Moses basket or cot drowsy but still aware (see 'Always Put Your Baby to Bed Aware', p. 94).

Listen to Your Baby

Crib Notes

- Take a moment to hear what your baby is saying when they cry.

- Stop, Listen, Look.

- Don't worry if you don't know what their cries mean. It takes time to know your baby.

- Some babies use noise as a way to settle themselves.

Babies don't come with a translation app (at least, not at time of writing) but over time, you will learn their language – long before they say their first words. We promise, no one is better placed to know what they need than you.

But how do you learn what they're trying to tell you? The only way is by listening and, as hard as it is, that means not rushing in to settle your baby too soon. There will always be an emotional response as a parent when you hear your baby crying. Mostly, it feels like they have a megaphone and are shouting 'Pick me up RIGHT NOW!' But their sounds can mean different things. And picking them up too quickly means not allowing yourself the opportunity to really hear them or for them to tell you what they need.

One of the useful things about having a routine is that it can help to translate what baby is saying and gives you your own personal guideline to connect their needs to their cry. As you get closer to a feed time, you'll hear baby's cry change and, suddenly, you'll have a lightbulb moment when you hear that cry again at a different time. Another cry that is quite distinctive and can be more recognisable than others is the overtired cry – but you're aiming not to get to that point!

Having said all this, don't be disheartened if you don't know the difference between their cries. You're learning a new language; some people study for months before they can even ask for '*dos cervezas por favor*'. Speaking Baby takes time.

Stop, Listen, Look

Studies have found our brains are hard-wired to have an instant reaction to a crying child. It triggers our fight-or-flight response, increasing our heart rate and pushing us into action.

A crying baby is not always a sad baby, though, which is worth remembering when it comes to sleep. Babies use cries to both process and communicate their emotions.

STOP

When you first hear your baby wake, it is natural to run to them, whether to get them up or to try to settle them before they fully wake. However, if you stop first and take a big breath, this will give you a moment to slow your heart to feel calm(er), which will help you to make a decision about what they are trying to tell you.

LISTEN

Listening helps you identify the different sounds your baby is making. Are they crying or babbling, or do they sound distressed?

Babies do make lots of different noises. If it's a low-level grumble, leave them and see how the sound develops. Once you have had a listen and you are confident your baby doesn't need you immediately, make yourself busy, as you're working against your caveperson instincts. We recommend making a cup of tea or going to the toilet; it's enough to distract you and it's a good amount of time to see if baby settles.

We know this is a difficult thing to do – we're hard-wired, remember? But we promise that starting to really hear your baby will help both of you in the long run (and not just where sleep is concerned).

Scale

The following is a communication scale. It's a guide for understanding your baby's noises, but we would recommend writing your own list, as only you know your baby's language.

- **1–3** These are grumbles, shouts and occasionally cries that can vary in sound and intensity but are largely content.
- **4** This is more of a whine. It is similar to a grumble, but mixed with the beginnings of more of a cry.
- **5** This is a 'cry-cry'. And usually indicates that they are hungry, overtired or overstimulated.

LOOK

If you have a video monitor or can see baby without them seeing you, check to see if their eyes are closed, they are moving their head side to side or rubbing their face? If so, it is likely to mean they are not happy to be awake yet and should be given a chance to go back to sleep without help from you.

Peak Before Sleep

Babies often make sounds as a way of settling themselves, and most will make some sort of noise before they go to sleep. Some babies will get even louder right before they go to sleep. We call this 'peak before sleep'.

For parents of peak before sleepers it can be confusing because picking them up can have the opposite effect and make babies more distressed when they were simply trying to go to sleep.

If you feel like your baby is not going to settle, give it another minute and see what happens. You will learn over time the sounds your baby makes when they are settling down for sleep.

SURVIVAL:
When your baby starts to make a noise, go for a pee before going to them; this will give you a chance to listen to their cry better.

MOVING FORWARDS:
Implement Stop, Listen, Look (see p. 61). Practise not rushing in and focus on whether they sound hungry, distressed or if they're just making themselves heard. Heads-up – this can be really hard at first!

Use Positive Sleep Associations

Babies might not talk but they use the same language of sleep as adults. Most of us have a pattern before we go to bed that helps get our brains into sleep mode: brush teeth, have a wee, put a glass of water (that you never drink) by the bed and read a book (like this one – but hopefully we're not sending you to sleep). We train our brains to know what happens next and we can do the same with our babies. Sleep associations are one of the most important parts of getting baby to sleep well.

Sleep Associations

If you use the same set of sleep associations consistently, in the same order, it tells your baby that it's time to sleep without using words.

- Put the lights on low to help the body to start producing melatonin, the hormone that signals it's time for sleep.
- Change baby's nappy so they are clean for sleep.
- Swaddle safely: swaddling prevents the startle reflex (which babies can have up until around 5 or 6 months); it helps them feel safe and secure and can even calm them down. Swaddle for all sleep, but make sure to unswaddle baby in between and for all feeds (see pp. 26–30).
- Swaddling isn't recommended if co-sleeping, so the sleep association then might simply be putting on a sleepsuit or pyjamas.
- Once weaned from a swaddle, a sleeping bag can also be considered a sleep association.
- Keep things calm and quiet.
- Use white noise.
- Soft singing or bedtime tunes can help because music triggers a part of the brain that can help you relax.
- Use special sleepy-time words as you put them down in the crib. These can be anything you feel comfy with, from 'night night' to a hopeful 'see you in the morning'.

Choose your sleep associations wisely. Cat learned the hard way that when she chose twerking, her baby seemed to be unable to sleep without it! And, unless you're a pop icon, it totally kills your back!

Sleep Comforters vs Sleep Props

There's a big difference between sleep comforters and sleep props. One is a useful tool that helps direct baby towards sleep, while the other is something that can be exhausting for a parent or caregiver.

What is a Comforter?

A comforter – such as a safe soft toy, muslin, breathable blanket or dummy or soother – can be an important sleep association for a child. It makes them feel safe and, generally, comforted. You are in control of baby's comforter. You may well be stuck with Mr Monkey for years! If you don't like a holey muslin or you don't want a thumb sucker, choose something else. Make sure it's safe for baby and, ideally, have more than one: one to keep, one to lose and one in a drawer for emergencies.

You also need to decide how you want to use a comforter. Is it for sleep only or is it something they can have with them at all times? And don't let other caregivers use it in a different way from you.

If your baby's comforter is a soft toy or blanket, sleep with it before giving it to your baby. It will make it smell of you and help to give even more comfort to baby when you're not there beside them. All our kids took their comforters with them when they went to nursery; this helped them settle there because it was like taking a bit of home with them.

What is a Sleep Prop?

A sleep prop is something baby cannot control on their own and, generally, requires a parent to be present, such as rocking, feeding to sleep or, sometimes, a soother or dummy. It's hard for baby to sleep well when these props become a habit as they require you or the prop to be there every single time they go back to sleep – which, if you think about the fact that a baby's sleep cycle is around 40–60 minutes, could be a lot.

Are Props Always Bad?

Some people love cuddling their baby to sleep. It's not a bad thing. In fact, there can be nothing better. However, it doesn't generally make for a restful night's sleep for parent or baby when it becomes something that happens every single time baby goes to sleep. Having said that, it is only a problem when it becomes a problem for you and your baby, and how rested you both are.

> *Sometimes you just need to do what you need to do. The idea is to have a structure and a foundation that you can come back to when you and baby are ready that will ensure a return to more restful sleep.*

Why is a Soother Both a Comforter and a Prop?

If you choose to use a soother (or dummy) as a comforter or sleep association, be aware that it might become a sleep prop. When babies are small, they suck a lot, so a soother can be a life saver. However, at the point when baby needs the soother to be replaced for all sleep, and cannot do so themselves, it becomes a prop, and you might want to think about exchanging it for something else or detoxing completely.

We recommend removing a soother before 6 months when babies have yet to fully understand object permanence, but tend to be less sucky. However, if you haven't managed it by then, do not worry. It is then better to keep it until baby can understand why you're taking it away, which will likely be closer to 2 years old.

How to Dummy Detox

The main reasons you might want to ditch the dummy are that your baby is waking frequently in the night and looking for it, they have other comforters and the dummy is no longer needed and/or they want the dummy all the time, not just when they are tired or going to sleep.

Follow these steps to detox:

- If you've been using the dummy throughout the day as well as during the night, start restricting the use to bedtime only, introducing something else if necessary, e.g. a breathable muslin or other comforter.
- After a few days of this routine and when you are comfortable and ready, take the dummy away completely.
- Once the dummy has been removed, use settling techniques for the first few days if needed – for example, hands-on comforting techniques (see p. 100).

Make sure that once you've decided to get rid of the dummy, you cut it up and put it in the bin, so you are not tempted to re-introduce it if you are having a bad night.

It's also ok to simply go cold turkey, if you wish.

A dummy or soother can be as much of a comforter to a parent as it is to baby. This can mean it is we who struggle saying goodbye more than they do! Once you have decided everyone is ready, commit to it. Your baby needs you to be consistent, so they don't get confused.

Age-appropriate Comforters

- **0–3 months:** swaddling (see p. 26)/gentle environmental changes for day and night/white noise (see p. 25)/dummy.
- **3 months:** swaddling/white noise/and you can introduce a comforter during feeds, so your baby gets used to seeing it and gives it a familiar smell.
- **4–6 months**: gently wean baby from swaddling (before they are rolling, for safety)/white noise/and you can introduce a comforter during feeds, so your baby gets used to seeing it and gives it a familiar smell.
- **6 months+:** the comforter can now be given to baby in their hands to allow them to use it as they wish. It can be introduced as a substitute for a dummy if you want to wean baby off using one.

SURVIVAL:

Sometimes you need to do what you need to do to get more sleep; but knowing how to change things when you are ready is key.

MOVING FORWARDS:

Be confident in making choices about your baby's sleep associations. You are in control of them. If you want to introduce something or take it away you can.

Be Consistently Consistent

Crib Notes

- Consistency is, perhaps, the most important rule of parenting.

- Your baby makes sense of the world by learning what happens next.

- There is no 'right' way; what matters is that your consistency works for you.

- Make a plan and trust yourself.

If you listen to our podcast, you will hear Sarah say 'consistency' about eleventy billion times. Well, at least she's consistent.

Babies and children understand the world through consistency; it helps them make sense of things. That doesn't mean there won't be slip-ups or changes, or that they don't need to learn to roll with things now and again. However, if you want your baby to do something every day, then you need to make sure *you* do the same things (almost) every day to achieve that. Consistency is, perhaps, the most important rule of parenting overall, not just for sleep.

Consistency might sound simple, but it's not. Parenthood is exhausting and sometimes the path of least resistance just seems easier. Being consistently consistent can be time-consuming because you need to make a plan. It can also require patience; you don't always see immediate results.

You need to be comfortable with your plan of action, bearing in mind the stage baby is at, how you are feeling and the support of those around you. Some parents can't cope with their baby crying for any longer than a minute; others can. There is no right way. However, all caregivers need to be on the same page of the bedtime story. Some babies find The Sleep Mums' Shoogle works (see p. 304), others the shush-pat. Only you know your baby. We hope to give you the tools and rules to find your own way.

The Sleep Mums' Rule of Three

In general, it takes around three days to establish a new habit for baby. Once your baby has shown you that they can do something for three nights (or days) in a row, that is your new normal. So, once you've done the hard work, stick to it.

If you haven't fed your baby at night for three nights, try not to slip back to it. But if you do, know that you have the tools to find your way back. If they've settled without your help, don't rock them to sleep again on the fourth day. If you have managed to get them to nap at the right times in the right place for half a week, keep going – you're an athlete, you've got this.

It's worth mentioning the three-day rule works the other way, too. Three days can be all it takes to go backwards or introduce a new, unwanted habit. It can then be even harder to go back to how it was before.

Changes will not always happen in three days, but it is usually a turning point and gives you something to focus on at the start. When you make a plan for change, you need to commit to it for at least three to five days, possibly up to a week or 10 days before you really see a difference, not succumbing for the odd nap here or there or a little sleep settling on the occasional night. You need to be consistent throughout that time. People often try something and then give up, saying that x or y doesn't work, when really they probably just gave up too soon.

We know it's hard, that's why we always recommend only making changes when you're ready.

So, work out the issue, with our help make a plan to change it and then phase the unwanted habit out – or, if you're ready, go cold turkey.

And always be consistent.

SURVIVAL:

Try to have a start time and an end time to your day. These two book ends will give you the most basic structure to base your day on.

MOVING FORWARDS:

What do you want your day(s) to look like? It doesn't need to be the same every single day, but make a plan, trust yourself and stick to it.

Have a Bedtime Routine

Crib Notes

- A bedtime routine signals it's time for the BIG sleep.

- Keep it simple.

- Focus on feeds and winding well.

- Consistency creates habit.

We know about the importance of sleep cues and associations as signals to sleep. And the bedtime routine is a massive sleep sign lit up in soothing neon lights.

It tells your baby that not only is it time to go to sleep, it's time to bed down for the 'big sleep'. Sleep associations are used for all sleep, but the bedtime routine is usually reserved for late afternoon, early evening. Many of the associations will be the same as for naps but it is useful to distinguish this sleep from the others, with a bath or massage and putting on a sleepsuit or pyjamas.

Massage is the rhythmic stroking of your baby's body. You can start at any age but when they are very small, they may find a long massage too stimulating.

One baby-massage technique might be gentle circles on their palms, feet or in a clockwise direction on their stomach (this one can help with digestion but use a light touch). You do not need to use oil.

Age-appropriate Bedtime Routines

There are no hard-and-fast rules for what your bedtime routine should look like. Some babies love baths, others don't. You do not need to include one in your bedtime routine if it will make everyone upset before you begin.

Your bedtime routine will have lots of the same elements as baby grows but start simple:

0–6 weeks

- In the very early days baby will not be able to cope with much more than a feed before bedtime.
- Small babies do not need to be bathed every day.
- A bath at bedtime can make baby too tired or too cold right before bed. If you want to bathe them, try doing it as an activity earlier in the day when they are less tired.
- Change baby's nappy and put on clean pyjamas to signal it's time for their long sleep.
- Milk feed. You want baby to have a really good feed at this time to make sure they sleep as long as they can. If

baby falls asleep when feeding, rouse them a little before putting them down.

- Wind thoroughly (see p. 33). Wind is never fun for baby, and you want to make sure there are no bubbles that can disrupt their sleep.
- Swaddle baby (see p. 26) after you have fed them.
- Turn on white noise (see p. 25).

2–4 months

- We recommend trying to avoid unplanned cluster feeding (see p. 44), so begin your bedtime routine by having two or more feeds close together, starting around 4pm for a 6/6.30pm bedtime.
- A warm bath or baby massage can help relax baby, but it can still be a lot for babies of this age. In place of a bath every day, top and tail and give baby a massage (see p. 75). Only use a product that you have tested on their skin previously.
- Change baby's nappy and put on clean pyjamas to signal it's time for their long sleep.
- Then another milk feed. You want baby to have a really good feed at this time to make sure they are satisfied. If baby falls asleep when feeding, rouse them a little before putting them down.
- Wind thoroughly (see p. 33). Wind is never fun for baby, and you want to make sure there are no bubbles that can disrupt their sleep.
- Swaddle baby (see p. 26) after feeding. If baby has started to roll, or you feel they are ready to stop being swaddled, follow our guide to gently stop using one (see p. 30).
- Turn on white noise (see p. 25).

- Start to use special sleepy-time words as you put them down, so creating another positive sleep trigger.

4–6 months

- Start by ending active play and put noisy toys away. Make this time calm and quiet.
- We recommend trying to avoid unplanned cluster feeding, so begin your bedtime routine with two or more feeds close together, starting around 4pm for a 6/6.30 bedtime.
- If you feel baby is too tired to take a full feed at 6.30, you can introduce a split feed, where they have half before bath or quiet time and the rest at bedtime. This works for breast or bottle.
- A warm bath or baby massage (see p. 75) can relax baby and help them to feel cosy and loved.
- Change baby's nappy and put them in clean pyjamas to signal it's time for their long sleep.
- Milk feed. You want baby to have a really good feed at this time to make sure they are satisfied. If baby falls asleep when feeding, rouse them a little before putting them down.
- Wind thoroughly (see p. 33). Wind is never fun for baby, and you want to make sure there are no bubbles that can disrupt their sleep.
- Put them in their sleeping bag before or after feed.
- Turn on white noise (see p. 25).
- Use special sleepy-time words as you put them down in the crib.

6 months+

- Start by ending active play and putting noisy toys away. Make this time calm and quiet.
- Once weaned, give baby their tea an hour before bath or massage, giving them time to digest it.
- A warm bath or baby massage (see p. 75) can relax baby and help them to feel cosy and loved.
- Once baby is established with solids, you can introduce a bedtime snack after bath or quiet time but before their milk feed (for example, cereal, rice or oatcakes or a banana; but try to avoid sugary fruits or snacks). This extra bit of food at bedtime can be useful when battling early wake-ups.
- Change baby's nappy and put them in clean pyjamas to signal it's time for their long sleep.
- Milk feed. You want baby to have a really good feed at this time to make sure they are satisfied. If baby falls asleep when feeding, rouse them a little before putting them down.
- Wind thoroughly (see p. 33). Wind is never fun for baby, and you want to make sure there are no bubbles that can disrupt their sleep.
- Put them in their sleeping bag before or after feed.
- Turn on white noise (see p. 25).
- Use special sleepy-time words as you put them down in the crib.

In the early days, giving baby a specific bed 'time' with a routine can seem a bit pointless. You know you're going to be seeing them long before morning. However, setting a bedtime routine early on helps you to be consistent as baby grows (it's also easier when you need to wrangle a toddler into a bath). Setting a baby's bedtime can also help you to have a little bit of an evening to yourself – to eat a meal, talk to your partner or even just go to bed early, too (as wild as that sounds).

SURVIVAL:
Keep it simple and consistent; feed, white noise and put them in their safe sleep environment.

MOVING FORWARDS:
Think about what you include in their bedtime routine so that it lasts. Try not to do anything now that you don't want to do as they get older.

Keep Night-time Calm and Fuss Free

Crib Notes

- Baby may need some noise to help them to sleep.

- White noise helps keeps the ambient noise consistent.

- Keep light and noise to a minimum.

- Be prepared for night feeds and nappy changes.

- Change a newborn nappy before a feed . . .

- . . . otherwise only change poo nappies.

- Be mindful of the midnight scroll.

Even the smallest amount of unfamiliar noise or stimulation can prevent baby from going to or staying asleep. Baby will be up for night feeds for at least the first few months, so make sure you keep all night feeds as calm and fuss free as possible.

Having said that, if baby was used to lots of noise when they were in the womb, you may find that they actually need some ambient noise to help them sleep. This is where white noise can be useful. Not only does the sound help baby to switch off but the whooshing sound imitates the noises they heard in the womb. It is also useful as a tool to keep the sound environment consistent for your baby, so they are less likely to be disturbed by a toilet flushing, noisy builders or the delivery guy.

Night Feeds, Not Night Club

Keep light to a minimum. You need to see what you're doing but not so much that it makes baby, or you feel like it's time to get up. Remember when we talked about jet lag and circadian rhythms in 'The First Two Weeks' (see p. 38)? Well, even as they grow night-time should feel like night-time.

Think about where you will feed at night. It's important to find a safe and comfortable place, where you won't fall asleep.

When you're exhausted, turning on the TV or a bright light to wake you up can feel like a good idea, but it can make it harder to go back to sleep afterwards. Use a small night light that gives you enough light to see your baby and get them to latch on to the breast or bottle well.

Make sure you have a drink nearby (if breastfeeding, a baby's latch can make your mouth drier than a badger's paw!) and maybe also a snack, in case you get the midnight munchies.

If you are combination- or formula-feeding, make sure you have bottles sterilised, and formula or breast milk easily to hand. Nobody needs to be clearing up (or crying) over spilt milk during the night.

Nappy Happy

Light and noise can overstimulate your baby at night, as can getting their nappy changed. The feelings, sensations, cooler air around their bum and seeing your lovely face right above them are like a full-moon party for your wee one.

Having everything set up for a nappy change helps. Use a small night light and make sure to have nappies, full change of clothes, wipes or cotton pads and water and changing mat nearby (often, it's easiest if the latter is on the floor by the bed).

Age-appropriate Guide to Night-time Calm

0–2 months

In the early days, when baby is up regularly for feeds, it's likely they will do more poos. In the first three months, check baby's nappy before a feed if they're not too hungry. This wakes them up and means you can change them if they have done a poo. If your baby tends to fall asleep easily while feeding, changing their nappy in the middle of a feed can be useful to wake them up and encourage them to take a full feed.

And as long as you haven't heard the distinctive rumble of the night train to Pooville, you'll then know they are clean when you put them down.

2 months+

Once they stop pooing as regularly overnight, you may find you do not need to change them at all at night. If they are regularly soaking through their nappy, go up a nappy or pad size for night-time (as long as the legs are snug) or look at different brands, which you may find work better for your baby.

If baby has bad nappy rash or any sores, change them more regularly.

As well as the stimulation, another reason for not changing them is that becoming dry at night (not having a pee when asleep) is a developmental milestone that baby is unlikely to reach for quite some time. So, if they're going to pee a lot at night, you don't want them to get into the habit of waking up to be changed. Especially when modern nappies are so efficient.

Over-stimulation for You

Waking up to feed your baby through the night is physically and mentally exhausting. In the same way that you're trying to keep things calm for baby, it's important to keep yourself calm, too.

Being up on your own and doing night feeds, it feels natural to reach for your phone, to scroll or connect with others, so you don't feel so alone. It can be a lifeline; but it can also have a negative effect on your headspace when your emotions are already stretched. Plus, the blue light from a phone can play havoc with your body clock. As an alternative, we can recommend a really good podcast about baby sleep to keep you company or some of our favourite audio books, like *Stepping Up* (The Unmumsy Mum), *Girl, Wash Your Face* (Rachel Hollis) and *Know Your Worth* (Anna Mathur).

SURVIVAL:
Be prepared and remember to look after yourself, too.

MOVING FORWARDS:
The calmer you can make night times, hopefully the calmer you will feel, and more able to make transitions when you and baby are ready.

Have a Breakfast Feed

> **Crib Notes**
>
> - **Awake associations help to create a waking habit.**
>
> - **Choose a time you want to get up.**
>
> - **Feed at that time every morning.**
>
> - **If baby is waking at a very early time, use techniques to gradually push towards the time you want their breakfast feed to be.**

Sleep associations help to get baby to sleep, but what we like to call 'awake associations' can help them to wake at roughly the same time each morning. One of the foundations of sleep is habit. We've talked about having a routine before bed: wash face, have a wee, set an alarm. But we also have them in the morning: unset alarm, have a wee, wash face. However, if you're a parent of a newborn, it's more likely to be: leap out of bed in a panic, run to crying baby, trip on a squeaky toy, curse, give dirty look to sleeping partner, apologise to baby for cursing.

But what if you could be baby's alarm clock, not the other way around?

We can't promise every wake-up will be as smooth as those before children, but you can gently encourage your baby to wake at a similar time every morning. Try giving your baby their first feed of the day (the 'breakfast feed') at the same time each morning. If you start and end your day at the same time each day, baby will learn this is the time to get up.

Unfortunately, it's not quite as simple as setting your alarm and choosing which perky song will wake you up. It can take time and patience. Your baby will need to be gradually edged towards the time that you want them to wake up. Their hunger can take time to catch on, too. The way to do it is by gradually distracting them for around 10 minutes every day from when they wake up until you feed them. This will allow you to get closer to the time you are aiming for. The idea is that by consistently feeding them at the same time, this will become the time they wake up and call for you.

So, if you would like baby to wake at around 7am and they are currently waking at 5.45am, it could take several weeks of slow adjustment and perseverance. Once your baby is able to go closer to 7am without a feed, always be consistent about feeding them at 7am (or as close to it as possible).

This guideline will only work if baby is getting the right amount of night sleep for them (10–12 hours). Sadly, you can't put baby to bed at 7pm and plan their wake-up for 9am. And putting baby to bed later doesn't mean they will automatically sleep later either. They like to keep you on your toes (literally).

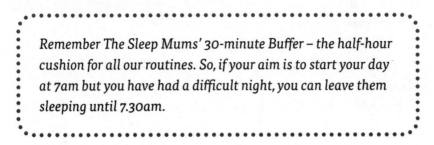

Remember The Sleep Mums' 30-minute Buffer – the half-hour cushion for all our routines. So, if your aim is to start your day at 7am but you have had a difficult night, you can leave them sleeping until 7.30am.

SURVIVAL:

Do not worry about this guideline too much if you are in survival. It is simply an idea that will help you to start your day with consistency and can be introduced at any point.

MOVING FORWARDS:

In The Sleep Mums' Rule of Three (see p. 72), we introduced you to the idea that most changes will start to happen in three days. With such gradual changes, achieving a set breakfast-feed time will take longer. Don't lose heart, though. A solid and consistent wake-up time is worth aiming towards as it helps to set up your day.

Don't Let Your Baby Get Overtired

Play is incredibly important, but babies can only cope with a short period of being awake before they need to go to sleep again. When baby gets overtired, cortisol and adrenaline are released into their bloodstream. These are wake-up hormones, not sleepy-time ones – and they make putting a baby to sleep much harder.

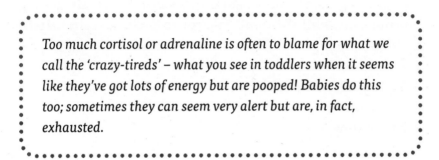

Too much cortisol or adrenaline is often to blame for what we call the 'crazy-tireds' – what you see in toddlers when it seems like they've got lots of energy but are pooped! Babies do this too; sometimes they can seem very alert but are, in fact, exhausted.

Here is an age-appropriate guide for how long baby can be awake:

Age	Awake Time
2–6 weeks	1 hour
6–12 weeks	1.5 hours (sometimes longer in the afternoon before bedtime)
3–4 months	1.5–2 hours (sometimes longer in the afternoon before bedtime)
4–6 months	2–2.5 hours (sometimes longer in the afternoon before bedtime)
6–10 months	2–2.5 hours, increasing to 3–3.5 hours in the afternoon as they get closer to 10 months

Remember that your baby's awake time always includes time for feeds. Even if they fall asleep in the middle of a feed, you want to wake them to finish it. If your 3-week-old wakes at 10am and feeds for an hour, they will need to go back to sleep almost straight after a nappy change around 11am. Not all babies will fall asleep easily, but it is much easier to settle one who still has energy to be settled than one who is overtired.

Overtired Signs (Not Just Your Eye Bags)

All babies are different, and their awake times will vary, but there are some signs that most babies will show if they are getting overtired. Knowing these will help you to read your baby better:

- Red-rimmed eyes
- Wide-eyed, frantic look
- Yawning
- Not settling

- **Turning head from side to side**
- **Rooting** (a reflex action where baby moves their head in the direction of touch and opens their mouth; it is often thought of as a 'feed-me cue' but doesn't always mean hunger)
- **Sucking fingers**

The last three also look like hunger signs, which is why you'll long to understand baby lingo. What makes it doubly hard is that feeding an overtired baby will lead to more wind and usually less sleep for everyone. That's one of the main reasons a routine is so useful, helping you to feel more confident that your baby's needs are fulfilled. Then, you know that when you see these signs, it's not because they're hungry.

If you feel your baby will not go to sleep after the above awake times, despite your best efforts, we recommend putting them down earlier, i.e. before you see these tired signs. They need energy to settle; getting them in the right environment for sleep for when they are tired is the easiest thing we can do to help them get there.

Overtired signs are especially useful for naps, as you may need to adjust the timings of your routine if you notice baby getting tired earlier. However, it's also helpful to look for them at the end of the day, as you edge towards bedtime and the bedtime routine. If you feel your baby is getting tired before you normally start to wind down, start the bedtime routine earlier. It can help relax them, prevent an overtired baby and a battle at bedtime.

A 'Window' to Sleep?

In the first five months, your baby will likely struggle to stay happily awake outside of their awake times – sometimes called awake windows – so you will find yourself adjusting naps and bedtimes, depending on how long they have been awake.

As they head towards the half-year mark, they will become more flexible with following a routine, even if they have been awake for longer than their 'window'. For example, if your 6-month-old's normal wake-up is 7am and they wake at 6am, you can still stretch them to their normal nap, therefore extending their awake time.

Too Much Fun?

Adults can become overwhelmed when there is too much noise, light, activity, people. And a baby's threshold is much lower, as their brain struggles to process it all, making overstimulation a surprisingly common problem.

Whereas we might use the excuse of needing to go to the toilet to get away from it all (just us?), a baby has no such option. When they become overstimulated they might start to show tired signs (see p. 88), become fussy or spaced out (like they are trying to zone out). It is your job to be their bathroom break before they get to that point. Take them away from the hubbub, cuddle them, allow them to snuggle into your shoulder and if you think they are tired, put them down for a nap.

Baby classes are a lifeline for many new parents, and we absolutely encourage you to go out and find one if you feel ready. Just be aware that an hour's class for a small baby is usually far too much for them to cope with.

The Witching Hour(s)

All babies have a time of the day, usually in the late afternoon before bedtime, when you may want to sell them on eBay. This is their Witching Hour(s) or, as we like to call it, the T/witching Hour(s) – when you keep twitching to check the clock to see if it's bedtime.

If a baby could talk during the T/witching Hour(s), they would probably say 'cuddle me, but don't touch me'. They need attention but are often too tired for it. It's pretty confusing for them – and for you!

T/witching Hour(s) can strike at any age, but are most common in the first few months or when baby is reaching new milestones, as they have been 'working harder' during the day to achieve skills. It's also likely that they've had their longest awake time in the second part of the afternoon.

So baby is tired, it's likely that you are tired (if breastfeeding, your milk supply may be lower at this time of the day) and family or partners may be coming back, making the home noisier and more overstimulating. There are two main ways to deal with these unmagical hours.

The first is food or milk; tiredness and hunger go together, which is something you can use to your advantage. They aren't interchangeable, but we can sometimes use food to fuel us when we are tired. This is why we recommend planning your cluster feeds in the early days (see p. 44) – this helps to fill baby up for the longer overnight sleep, while also giving them energy to make it through to bedtime. As they get older and are weaned you can use a 'supper' as an extra meal to help them if they are very tired.

The second way to help is to distract them as much as possible – go for a short walk (so they don't fall asleep!) or start their bedtime routine earlier and take longer with the calming elements, like baby massage (see p. 75).

> *It might be something more than a bit of witchcraft causing your baby's unsettledness – say, reflux or another digestive issue. These can be more common at night; but if your baby is content most of the time then cries inconsolably in the late afternoon and evening, it could be a case of the twitching.*

Touched Out?

Feeling 'touched out' is when parents (and babies) reach a point where they become averse to physical contact and want a kind of time-out for their bodies. It is often a reaction to overstimulation. It can feel like your skin is itching, the room is closing in or you may feel anger or nausea at the thought of being touched by another human.

It is normal. Fulfilling your baby's needs can be physically and mentally exhausting, and often your body is at the centre of fulfilling those needs. If you have to take time out, it does not make you a bad parent or partner. And if you think your baby might be feeling touched out, don't be afraid to put them down somewhere safe and give them some space, too. You can stay beside them but give both of your bodies a rest.

SURVIVAL:
Respond to their cues and be aware of their feed times.

MOVING FORWARDS:
Establish a more structured routine so that you can make plans around meeting baby's needs.

Always Put Your Baby to Bed Aware

Crib Notes

- Practise putting your baby to bed so they are aware of their surroundings from birth.

- You are not a ninja: the arm transfer is too hard to perfect.

- They need to be relaxed going to sleep where they are going to stay

- Use winding (see p. 33) as a technique to ensure you put them down aware but not fully awake.

- Don't assume that they won't be able to do it.

This is the guideline that can drive parents loopy because it sounds counterintuitive. However, it is one of the most significant as baby grows: they need to be relaxed falling asleep where they are going to stay for the nap or night, otherwise, it's likely they won't stay there very long.

You might have heard people talk about putting baby into their cot awake, but we feel this is a little misleading. It suggests to parents that their baby should be going to bed bright-eyed and ready for a peek-a-boo party. If your baby has started to drift off in your arms, you do not need to wake them up fully – rather, it is making sure that they are aware of their surroundings that is really important. This is why we like to say you should put baby into their cot *aware*.

In the first few weeks and months, as you and your baby are getting to know one another and settling into a routine, putting baby to bed asleep is an easy thing to do. They are usually more tired and less likely to notice a change in scene. But when a 2–3-month-old baby falls asleep in your arms and you put them down in their cot, it can be disorientating for them. (Imagine going to sleep in your bed, then waking up in the living room.) They expect you to still be there – which is why they can get very upset when they wake – and be much harder to settle afterwards.

Full disclosure: both of us have cuddled our babies to sleep, especially when they were newly minted. But while it's hard to resist the occasional newborn snuggle, we still recommend practising getting baby down aware of their surroundings. It's worth bearing in mind, though, that if you are not putting them down aware and sleep suddenly gets trickier, this could be the reason why. Around half of the parents that Sarah sees find that sleep improves immediately just following this one guideline.

At night, a great way to ensure baby still goes to bed drowsy but aware is by winding them thoroughly (see p. 33) – it rouses them just enough.

Another problem is that the arm-to-cot transfer does not work every time. Your baby might have been sleeping soundly in your arms, but you wake them with a jolt because your hand has gone to sleep. This pain in the arm can lead to bigger ones – bellowing tears from baby and having to start the sleepy-time routine all over again.

As a parent or caregiver, you take baby to the edge of sleep with your bedtime routine and sleep associations (see pp. 74 and 64). Allowing them to fall asleep by themselves aware of their surroundings helps during all subsequent wake-ups; baby feels comfortable going back to sleep where they are because they've already done it.

SURVIVAL:

When you are just trying to make it through, it's ok to put baby to bed asleep; just be mindful of the impact it can have on sleep overall.

MOVING FORWARDS:

Once you've made the decision to put them down to bed aware, they might go to sleep themselves, but you may also need to start implementing techniques in the cot or sleep space to help them.

Learn How to Settle Your Baby

Babies learn so much in the first year of life. Walking, talking, eating and, of course, doing the Hokey Cokey . . . These skills are not all automatic – even the things our bodies do naturally can take patience and practice to do well.

As parents, we guide babies through learning things, from holding their hands as they totter on tippy-toes to playing aeroplanes with a spoon when they are weaning. And yet, folk often get a hard time for wanting to help their baby to sleep. But enabling them to get good sleep is one of the most valuable things you can do for them – and you. It affects everything from their development to their mood.

'Cry it out' and 'controlled crying' are horrible phrases and leave most parents shuddering in their exhausted slippers. But helping your baby to sleep better doesn't have to mean leaving them to cry for hours on their own.

What is Settling?

Settling is a broad term, covering self-settling and assisted settling.

Self-settling

Self-settling is as it sounds: when your baby can manage to get off to sleep without any (or minimal) help from you. It's important to understand your own expectations when it comes to self-settling. Teaching a baby to fully soothe themselves is usually a long and non-linear process (and why you'll still be cuddling your 18-year-old after a heartbreak).

Assisted Settling

Assisted settling (or nurturing settling) is finding something that works for you and your baby to help them sleep.

This kind of settling requires consistency and perseverance on your part. There are lots of different techniques, but the key thing with gentle assisted settling is that if you want your baby to settle in the cot, you comfort them until fully asleep to start.

Then you gradually stop using the settling technique before they are fully asleep and, finally, only use it until they are calm.

Settling Techniques

Settling will mean different things for different babies and parents. It's important to find the thing that works for you.

Remember: settling techniques should be used at every settle.

There are a number of ways to settle your baby gently – some as simple as using the sleep associations you have used at bedtime (see p. 64), others requiring a more hands-on approach:

- The Sleep Mums' Shoogle (see Glossary, p. 304)
- Tummy rubbing
- Hand holding
- Face rubbing
- Bottom patting
- Back rubbing
- Supported tummy with bottom patting – use one arm under baby under their hips, lift slightly and use the other hand to pat their bottom (it may sound like you need to be made of arms to make this work but once you get the hang of it, it can be a really good way to settle baby – especially if they're used to you patting their bottom when in your arms or they have started standing in the cot)

As your baby develops, techniques that previously worked can stop working and you may end up climbing the walls as they try to climb out of the cot.

If baby is standing, let them stand and you kneel or stand next to the cot with your arms around them letting them cuddle in, allowing you to rub their back or pat their bottom until they relax, ready to be laid down. You may need to repeat this process multiple times to get baby to sleep and use the supported-tummy-with-bottom-patting technique.

Back to Settling

Babies should always be put down on their backs to sleep. Some babies like to be settled on their tummy with a back or bottom pat or using The Sleep Mums' Shoogle (see Glossary, p. 304) but you can roll them over once they are calm. Depending on their age, and if they are able to safely roll from back to front and front to back, they may find their own sleeping position on their tummy. Check out the Lullaby Trust (see Resources, p. 305) for full safe-sleeping guidelines.

Talking Baby

As you progress with listening to your baby (see p. 60), you will start to recognise the different sounds they make. At first, you might want to pick them up at every peep, but as you start to learn that they are ok and not always needing you right this second, you will feel more comfortable in leaving them.

With all our gentle settling techniques there will likely still be some tears, but the key thing is you are not leaving baby alone. You are giving them comfort and assistance to get to sleep.

You will learn the different sounds your baby makes – which ones mean what and when to react. The fastest way to work this out is by following Stop, Listen, Look (see p. 61) and keeping a note of your baby's cries.

Sleep Settling by Age

Helping baby to learn the skill of sleep can be as simple as setting up great sleep habits and teaching them to settle themselves. But not always. So, what do you do when your baby is solidly in a routine and takes good, full feeds, but still wakes frequently at night or during naps?

The really important part of settling baby is being completely consistent in your approach, using the same settling techniques with your sleep associations every time. 'Be consistently consistent' is probably Sarah's most-used phrase, but it is key to baby sleep.

Age-appropriate Settling Guidelines

The following are age-appropriate settling guidelines. However, some babies will be able to settle themselves earlier than others, and some parents may feel more comfortable in using settling techniques sooner.

0–2 months
In the first couple of months, feed as much as you want to settle your baby when they need comfort.

2–4 months

When baby wakes, allow them to fuss and grumble for a short while before getting up to go to them. This allows you a moment of breathing space to hear what kind of cry they are making. This gets easier as baby gets older and you get to know each other better: are they hungry, in distress or coming out of a deeper phase of sleep and not happy about it? (Basically, us on a Monday morning.) You may find that your baby settles after a few cries. It can be important to leave them for a few moments, so you don't disturb their own process of moving between sleep cycles.

If baby continues crying, check on them and put back in place one or two of the sleep associations you have used in their bedtime routine, like white noise, 'shushing' or their comforter (see p. 66). Then leave their cribside or room. Your baby may now settle.

If not, baby may be looking for a little comfort, so before you lift them up, which might disturb them further, use gentle to firm pressure with your hand on their chest or gently massage the left side of their tummy for digestion. This is a gentle introduction to the No-lift Settle (see p. 104).

If baby still doesn't settle and you're confident that you've tried everything, you can offer them a feed.

4–6 months

When baby is a little bit older, you will be beginning to learn their language and may feel more comfortable in knowing why they are crying. Try to leave them a little longer to hear what their cry is telling you. If baby continues to cry at the same level continuously, return and try the No-lift Settle (see p. 104).

6 months+

There are a lot of changes around 6 months. Baby will have started solids, they may be sleeping in their own room, and napping and moving around more. It can be a lot for them to cope with, so be gentle with any big sleep changes around now.

Make sure you and baby are in a comfortable routine with any daytime changes before you start looking at night settling. You'll often find that the daytime changes will make a big difference, once they are used to them. Always allow three to five days for day routines to become the norm.

When you feel comfortable and ready, you can look at sorting out night sleep. Once you do, make sure everyone in the family is on board and committed to settling in the ways we've described. It can be hard work for several nights, so partners and other caregivers need to be able to give support and settle baby in exactly the same way.

The No-lift Settle

Find a part of baby's body that you can rub or pat to soothe them and 'shush' loudly, recreating a sound similar to white noise. This reminds them that you're there and takes their mind off crying. The aim is to get them to calm down, then become drowsy and, ultimately, fall asleep. You need to pat or rub quite firmly to achieve a soothing distraction. Then gradually slow down the 'shush', rub, pat or 'The Sleep Mums' Shoogle' as baby settles, until you are barely doing anything at all. Always finish by stopping the movement with your hand and letting the weight of it comfort baby for a few moments before removing it entirely. Then, without making a big deal of it, leave the cotside or room.

Your baby may cry a little, but that's to be expected. If they do, give them a little while to try to settle themselves after you've left. Try to listen to their cries and then, when you feel you need to, go back in and resettle them in their cot again.

Repeat until baby settles.

Settling a baby in this way will take longer on the first night, but if you commit to doing it in the same way every night, they will gradually need your help less and less. The age of your baby, how often they are up during the night and how long the sleep issues have been going on, will dictate how long it takes. In general, though, it is likely to take three to five nights of settling like this before they will begin to do it on their own.

It can feel hard doing the No-lift Settle. When Cat was first trying out this technique, I reminded her that when she was walking her daughter round the block to sleep, she would still cry. It just doesn't feel as horrible because you are outside in the fresh air and doing something active to help your baby sleep. The No-lift Settle is a lot like walking your baby in the early days; you are helping them to sleep, even if it doesn't feel like it. But we promise, you are.

Settling Tips

- Set goals and stick to them. If you've decided you want baby to have comfort from you but ultimately self-settle, then you need to give them a chance. That means leaving them to try.
- If you need a break, it's ok to have one – and let baby cry a little. This does not make you a bad parent.
- Tag team with a partner or family member if it gets too much.
- White noise and 'shushing' need to be louder than you think.

If you feel your attentiveness is agitating and overstimulating your baby – which is more common than you may think – then it's better to leave them to try to settle on their own.

> *Your baby's cries can sound like a siren in your heart. It's one of the hardest parts of settling, especially if they're overtired, when they can sound frantic, making you want to react immediately, hoiking them up and holding them close. There is nothing wrong with this innate response, but it's worth remembering that sometimes your baby is crying because they want to be asleep and by picking them up, you can stop them doing so and prevent their natural sleep pattern from progressing.*

A Word on Wind

Wind is often the thing that wakes babies up with a sudden painful cry, any time from shortly after going to bed to later on during their nap or at night. If you suspect baby has wind when you go in to resettle them, pick them up and try to get a burp out of them (see p. 33) before attempting to use your settling techniques.

SURVIVAL:

Try some settling when your baby wakes, but don't feel you have to persevere until they go back to sleep. You might get a win sometimes, which will boost your confidence and might get you to the point where you are ready to move forwards.

MOVING FORWARDS:

If baby is waking through the night, try to use the settling techniques you have found to work for them to extend the times between wake-ups and/or feeds, depending on their age.

Have a Daytime Routine

We truly believe that, ultimately, having a routine allows you to be more flexible, not less. If baby and you know what should be happening in your 24 hours, everyone will be happier.

The key to a good routine is keeping it simple. And you will see that each of our routines builds on the one before, which means you don't have to completely relearn a new routine every few months. Once you get the hang of it, you'll be surprised that it will become second nature for both you and baby.

If you always eat lunch at 12pm, your stomach will start rumbling at 11.59am. It already knows it's lunchtime. Doing things at roughly the same time every day is a good thing for adults – and it's definitely a good thing for babies. They don't know a lot about the world, but the cosy embrace of a routine and knowing what comes next makes them feel safe. It's also good for their cognitive development; they need time to sleep and process all they've learned.

What is a Routine?

A routine is a predictable pattern that is easy for you to follow. It takes the guesswork out of wondering if baby is hungry or tired, which can be hard in the early days when you're getting to know them. It also helps parents know if something is up – for example, if their baby's eating is out of whack. A routine directed by you and not by baby is one that you can control and is largely consistent, meaning baby becomes familiar with feed, sleep and play patterns, giving them a feeling of security and comfort.

What is Not a Routine?

A routine does not mean you cannot go out, go to parties, take your other child to nursery or have family dinners. It does not have to be a prescriptive, clock-based regime. An army sergeant is not going to make you do press-ups if baby does not do X at 7.47am. Nor will your whole day be a write-off.

What You Need to Fit into A Day

The important part of a routine is making sure you meet your baby's needs through sleep, feeds and active and quiet time. To start with, that covers a 24-hour period. Once they are big enough, the active part of the routine is confined to their daytime hours, generally between 7am and 7pm (or the times you want your 12-hour day to start and end).

We like to think of the parts of a routine as the foundations of your day that you can build on, but without worrying about the whole thing crashing down if you don't do all of them. Every. Single. Day. If there are days when your routine doesn't work, don't worry.

Under the Weather

It's normal to worry when your baby isn't feeling well about how it will affect their routine. A change in sleeping and eating can be the first signs that something is up. It's important to remember that babies will often feel comforted by keeping their routine as normal as possible. Don't be afraid to follow their needs and cues, too, though, which may be different when they aren't feeling themselves, and use The Sleep Mums' 30-minute Buffer (see p. 35) as much as you need to cover disrupted naps or bad nights. If they are looking for more feeds, for thirst or comfort, give it to them, unless a medical professional has recommended otherwise. Babies can also go off their milk or food when they don't feel right, but continue to offer it to them as usual. And finally, if you and baby want to take a duvet day and forget about routines and what should be happening when, that is ok. You have the knowledge and skills to make things better when you are both feeling it.

If you are ever concerned about your baby's health, always call or go and see a doctor. Trust your instincts. You know your baby best.

What Your Baby Needs by Age

Here is a breakdown of what your baby's day might look like from birth to 12+ months.

Birth–2 Weeks

- **Feeds & Sleep** Baby will be feeding roughly every 2–2.5 hours (so 12+ feeds in 24 hours) and napping in between, day and night.
- **Play** When a baby is small, you are their greatest toy. However, at first, this can be a bit overwhelming. It doesn't always come naturally. The best thing to remember is to keep it simple. This is especially true when they are new, as they will easily become overstimulated.

2–8 Weeks

- **Feeds & Sleep** Your baby will be feeding roughly every 2–3 hours (around 10 feeds in 24 hours) and having around six naps during the day, then overnight sleep.
- **Play** For a newborn, even changing their nappy can feel like playtime. There are lots of sensory experiences involved and usually their caregiver's lovely face is leaning over them. Faces are really exciting to babies. They love to look at you and watch how your face moves when you talk to them.

Babies find out about the world through what they can see, hear, touch, smell and taste. So, whether that's a squeaky toy or a black-and-white book, it's as exciting as watching Netflix is to us.

You can start practising short periods of tummy time from birth and build up to longer sessions as they get more comfortable, looking like they're attempting to swim on dry land!

Don't feel you have to 'play' with your baby. Your love and attention, your cuddles and care will often be enough to entertain them.

8–16 weeks

- **Feeds & Sleep** Your baby will be feeding roughly every three hours (8–10 feeds in 24 hours) and they may do slightly longer stretches at night. They will be having around four to five naps during the day, then overnight sleep.
- **Play** Now it's time to get more serious about playtime. At this stage, you want baby to be spending more of their playtime on their stomach. Lying on their tummies prepares babies for exploring the world on their own. Daily practice helps develop a strong neck and core.

  From a sleep point of view, tummy time is important because when they wriggle about it helps to dislodge wind, meaning better sleep. And stronger neck muscles help baby to feed better, also meaning sounder sleep.

  It's not just tummy time that helps with sleep at this age. Taking time to play on the floor or on a play mat with baby looking up at the ceiling encourages them to feel more comfortable in a safe back-sleeping position and helps to stretch their little bodies out.

4 months

- **Feeds & Sleep** By this stage, your baby will feed three-hourly during the day, plus any feeds overnight. They will have approximately four daytime naps, then overnight sleep.
- **Play** By the time babies are reaching out and grasping for things, a whole new level of baby play has arrived. They may finally be able to shake that rattle that Auntie Ali got them when they were born. And they'll enjoy discovering textures and more in the way of sensory play.

  They're also likely to be more engaged in your facial expressions.

5 months

- **Feeds & Sleep** By 5 months, we recommend baby feeds at approximately 7am, 10am, 12.15pm, 3pm, 5pm, 6.30pm, plus any overnight on a 7am–7pm routine. We group feeds together before a long nap and bedtime to help baby sleep (see p. 44). They will have approximately three day naps, then overnight sleep.
- **Play** When babies start to move on their own it brings more exciting play (and, usually, more worry!). Rolling, reaching and grasping allow them to make things happen by themselves. It's their first taste of independence. At this age, parents or caregivers should show them how to do things, but also to give them the (safe) space to start to try things themselves.

  If baby is actively rolling and pushing up by themselves, think about the safety of their sleep set-up (see 'Your Sleep Tool Kit', p. 20).

6–9 months

- **Feeds & Sleep** When baby has weaned, their day feeds will usually have evolved into four main feeds during the day. Their day sleep will also have consolidated into two slightly longer naps.
- **Play** From 6 months, your baby's play will develop into more complex games. They'll love watching you building towers and knocking them down; at this age, cause and effect is a big source of enjoyment.

  So is making a lot of noise. If you've always wanted to be in a band, now's the time; musical instruments will be a big hit. Or just be your baby's groupie and listen as they play.

  Sensory play is also worth getting stuck into at this age – different textures, shapes and smells will captivate your baby. Socialising becomes more important, too, so if you've not made it to any baby classes yet, looking for a local playgroup can be useful. But you are enough for your baby if you're not ready to socialise.

9–11 months

- **Feeds & Sleep** Between 9 and 11 months, as they eat more solid food, baby will drop another of their day feeds, bringing it to three. They will continue with two naps and overnight sleep.
- **Play** Baby will be getting more adventurous both in play and exploration. They might be crawling or even walking. A lot of babies at this age like to pull themselves on to their knees and do a little wiggle. This movement helps with hip mobility, which is vital for walking.

  Now that they're older, messy play is a great way to muck about. It might feel like you're already spending most of your day clearing up after your little one, but getting grubby together can be surprisingly liberating and an amazing way for them to learn.

> *We have a saying: 'if in doubt, go out'. The world is baby's playground. A walk in the fresh air can be a game changer if you're struggling to know what to do. It blows away bad moods and is a rich source of things to look at and talk about.*

11–12 months

- **Feeds & Sleep** By the time they reach their first birthday, most babies will be down to approximately two feeds a day and two naps, and hopefully getting a full night's sleep.
- **Play** Your baby will now likely be communicating more and showing you emotions. This unlocks another level of play. They will delight in showing you toys and they may be able to follow simple instructions. They will love looking at things with you and books will become increasingly valuable.

12 months +

- **Feeds & Sleep** From this age onwards, some babies will continue to have milk at breakfast and bedtime, others will not. As long as they are eating a good, varied diet you can be led by them. Most babies will drop to one longer nap, usually after lunch, between 14 and 16 months, but it can happen as early as 12 and as late as 18 months.
- **Play** Your baby will be getting better at using their hands and fingers and will probably be feeding themselves with

their fingers at most meals. This means you need to keep an eye on small toys and keep them out of reach. Messy play with food that they can eat, though, can be another great game to add into your day.

Another milestone is that as their strength grows with walking and standing, they might start to dance or bop along to music. People talk about dad dancing, but baby dancing is the ultimate!

SURVIVAL:

If you don't follow a routine, try to write things down and see if you already have one. This can be as simple as a few hooks to hang your day on, so you and your baby know what is happening next. Then, when you feel ready, you can start to implement more structure.

MOVING FORWARDS:

Once you feel confident with your routine, you may feel ready to be more flexible and even start to hack it on some days (see 'Hack a Routine', p. 117).

Hack a Routine: Making It Work For You

Crib Notes

- **One routine will never fit everyone every day.**

- **Routines are not for every parent . . .**

- **. . . but if you want to see results, don't give up on them too soon.**

- **Your baby's needs in 24 hours are sleep, feeds and active and quiet time . . .**

- **. . . how you shape how that looks is up to you, as long as those needs are met.**

- **Remember The Sleep Mums' 30-minute Buffer for all our routines (see p. 35).**

A lot of parenting advice seems to forget that one size of routine is never going to fit all. It doesn't take into account a partner's work hours, childcare hours, nursery times, a preference for a longer morning nap, baby yoga (get you!), siblings or that your little one was up and down like a pogo stick last night. This simplistic approach leads parents to feel that a routine is too restrictive.

The other reason why parents say routines don't work is because they can't make them fit with their own existing routine. When they're exhausted and struggling to even make a cup of tea (then drink it), it can make them feel like they've failed. Not so good for the old parenting morale. So, they chuck out the idea of routine altogether.

Hacking a Routine to Meet Your Baby's Needs

In 'Have a Daytime Routine' (see p. 108), we spoke about what baby needs in a 24-hour period. But it's unrealistic to expect a routine to work for you every single day – things come up and you and baby need to feel comfortable with being flexible – and with some guidance, fitting baby's needs into a day can be shaped more by you.

Firstly, all our routines have a half-hour buffer throughout the day. You may find you only use this once or twice in a day but it's there to give you a little flexibility if you need it. We realise that might not feel like much, given how complicated many people's lives are. But it can be helpful to stop you feeling like you're always clock-watching and empower you to watch your baby instead.

You might also choose to consistently shift the start and end time of your day. We talk about 7am–7pm because this generally works for baby as they grow. Once they start going to regular nursery and then school, they will likely have to be up by around 7am. Getting kids to bed early (around 7pm) is also beneficial as it works with their natural circadian rhythm, stops them getting overtired and can give you a break.

At the end of this chapter, you'll find a few routine-hack examples. But now, without further ado . . .

Feeds

- **Milk** Babies need to eat very regularly, so while the exact time of the feed may vary, this is one thing that has to stay fairly consistent, especially when they are new, as it will need to be close to every two hours. You can usually feed baby 30 minutes before a feed is due, and some (but not all) can stretch to 30 minutes after it's due. As they get older, though, they will gradually become more flexible.
- **Solids** When you are weaning baby on to solids, you will need to fit meals into your day around milk feeds and nap times. Meals can be a little flexible to allow eating together with family, if that matters to you. The most important thing is that baby is not too tired or too hungry to enjoy eating. We all know what hangry (see Glossary, p. 302) looks like – and it ain't pretty.

Sleep

- **Naps** The point of napping is to prevent your baby getting overtired. So, while the exact times and lengths of naps can be flexible, you always need to bear this in mind when looking at baby's day.

  Another point to note if adapting one of our routines is that your baby's last nap should not fall too close to bedtime.
- **Night sleep** The reason that most folk choose to start the day between 6 and 7am is because that is what works for parents returning to work and, ultimately, for the child when they go to nursery, then school.

It is possible to shift the whole routine – for example, if you want your family to have dinner at 6 or 7pm, you can push bedtime closer to 8 or 8.30pm using an 8am–8pm routine. It doesn't always follow that baby will sleep later in the morning, but you can aim to make up the difference in naps (or bring their first nap earlier) if they are tired.

> *You are aiming for a 10–12-hour stint in bed. Nobody sleeps through the night without waking, but most of us stay in bed (and even believe we stay asleep) overnight for one long sleep.*

Love, Play and Interaction

Play and attention are really useful tools; they can be excellent distractions when you are trying to encourage baby to stretch between milk feeds or make it through to sleep time if you have hacked a routine or things are just not going to plan.

Remember, though, a baby's idea of play is different to ours. The world is literally their playground. So, any play or attention must be age-appropriate (see pp.111–116) – because an overstimulated baby can easily become tired and cranky.

> *Hacking a routine is not just about the timings of baby's sleep; it's also about how feeds and active time interact with their sleep.*

Routine Hacks

It can be easier to start your day with a routine change, rather than trying to add it in later. For example, waking earlier to give baby a feed at 6.30am, which then shifts your day back. Or, alternatively, distracting them, so their first feed is at 7.30am, so shifting the day forwards. This can give you more flexibility later in the day.

Here are some examples of how you could hack our routines.

Q. My baby has swimming on a Monday at 10, but that's when she is due a feed. What should I do?

A. If you can walk to your class, use the walk as a time for her nap and then arrive slightly early so you can feed baby before class. Or distract them in the morning so that they take a slightly later feed at 7.30, meaning your next feed will be at 10.30am.

Q. My baby has yoga at 2pm, but that coincides with her long nap. Can I go?

A. Of course! But try a slightly earlier nap on that day and be prepared that baby may not last to the end of the class without a top-up feed to keep them going. They may also need a catnap on the way home, but if bedtime is 7pm, try not to let this be any longer than 15 minutes, if they've had a good earlier nap, or any later than 3.30pm.

Q. My 9-week-old baby woke at 4.30am and slept until 8am and now my day is out of whack. I have a class at 1.30pm. Should I miss it or can I hack back on track?

A. Aim for a nap at 9.30–10.30, then feed baby when they wake. Afterwards, pop them in the pram to walk to your class or in the car and let them sleep en route. Offer another feed at 1pm, ahead of your class together. On the way home, they may nap again, then feed at 4pm and you are back on track for your age-appropriate bedtime routine.

SURVIVAL:

For some people, survival will be sticking to a routine; for others, it might be not starting one until they are ready. You do you.

MOVING FORWARDS:

Pick a day and choose something out of the ordinary that you'd like to do. It might be a class or a lunch out with friends. Write down how you could change your routine to make sure you fit in everything your baby needs at this stage. Then go for it!

Wake Your Baby From Naps to Keep Routine

Crib Notes

- Day sleep is as important as night sleep.

- Be consistent with naps now, to allow you more flexibility later.

- Did we mention be consistent?

- Try not to let baby get overtired.

- DO wake a sleeping baby to stick to a routine.

- Know your danger nap.

Parents often focus on night-time sleep because that is when we all want to get some shut-eye. However, the better babies sleep during the day, the better it will usually be at night. Naps are an essential part of the lives of happy and contented babies and parents, so we feel they should be guarded as closely as the last biscuit in the tin.

We recommend trying to stay at home for at least one nap and putting baby to bed in the same place that they sleep at bedtime when you are trying to establish a routine. The reason is that they are likely to have a better, more solid sleep in their bed with little or no external distraction, than they would in the buggy or elsewhere. This doesn't need to be every day, just most.

At times it might feel frustrating or isolating to be at home when baby is napping. However, you know those old ladies who tell you it goes too quickly? Well, that generally goes for the tough stuff, too. You only have to be absolutely consistent with your nap routine for a fairly short time. In fact, the more adjusted your child is in a routine, the easier it is to be flexible on odd days.

We have all seen or heard about parents running around, rocking baby, bouncing baby, driving baby (and themselves) bonkers trying to get them to sleep. It might help once or twice, but in the long term, the only thing that will consistently get baby to sleep is being consistent. Naps, like bedtime, need their own routine and sleep associations.

> How well your baby goes down for their nap depends on how long they've been awake. It's much harder to get an overtired baby to nap well. It's one of the reasons we recommend a routine – it helps you have a better idea of whether baby is tired, hungry or wants to play.

When to Nap

Your baby's naps will change almost as much as they do during the first year.

While each baby is different, they usually have similar sleep patterns, depending on their stage and age. By the time they get to 4–6 months, most babies will be on around three naps a day, before dropping down to two between 6 and 8 months, then one between 12 and 16 months.

> *The morning nap is often the easiest for baby to settle into,*
> *even though they have often just had a longer sleep overnight.*
> *One reason could be that they are not overtired. And it's*
> *almost like they think, Oh yes, sleep. I quite like this!*

Following a nap routine can be really useful, but also look to your baby for sleep cues and remember you can be flexible by half an hour. This adjustment is worth remembering if you miss a nap or baby struggles to sleep, and you may need to bring the next nap or bedtime forwards.

When Not to Nap

As much as it's important to get baby to nap at the right time, it's also really important to wake them to keep to your routine. We know this goes against every fibre of your sleep-depleted being. But if you let baby sleep for too long during the day, they are likely to wake up more regularly or be awake for longer at night.

Another reason to wake baby from a nap is if it's getting too close to bedtime. If you are following a routine (natural or planned), once baby has dropped their third nap, we don't recommend napping after around 3.30pm as this can become a danger nap.

Danger Nap

This is a late nap that happens close to bedtime. A danger nap can be as little as 4 minutes that can add 40 minutes to your bedtime routine because baby will not settle as easily. You want to make sure your baby has had good naps earlier in the day, which may involve resettling them, so they can make it through to bedtime without taking a danger nap.

Power Naps vs Danger Naps

When is a power nap a danger nap? A power nap is the shorter, end of the day nap that you can have in your parenting pocket to crack out when needed. At first, it is a necessity; but by the end of baby's first year it stops being so useful because it is more likely to be a danger nap.

Age-appropriate Guide to Power Naps

- **0–4 months** Baby will have four clear naps.
- **4–5 months** Baby will have three clear naps.
- **5–6 months** By this age, the third nap is moving towards a power nap and you should keep it to 20–30 minutes.
- **6–7 months** Baby will have two clear naps but may need a power nap (10–20 minutes) on the odd day.
- **7 months+** This is when a power nap can slide into the danger-nap zone and should be used in emergencies only.

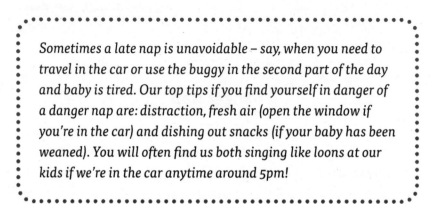

Sometimes a late nap is unavoidable – say, when you need to travel in the car or use the buggy in the second part of the day and baby is tired. Our top tips if you find yourself in danger of a danger nap are: distraction, fresh air (open the window if you're in the car) and dishing out snacks (if your baby has been weaned). You will often find us both singing like loons at our kids if we're in the car anytime around 5pm!

SURVIVAL:
Focus on getting the naps, not how you get them.

MOVING FORWARDS:
Be consistent with how you want naps to look and aim to get at least one at home as you focus on establishing a nap routine.

Nap on The Go
(but not all the time)

Crib Notes

- Do go out for some naps.

- Use the same sleep associations as at home.

- Baby might sleep less soundly out and about.

- You might need to bring the next nap or bedtime forwards if they become overtired.

- There is a 30-minute buffer on all our routines (see p. 35).

- One bad nap will *not* create unwanted sleep habits.

A lot of other books and parenting advice will tell you your baby must sleep at home for all naps, so you don't miss a single one. However, we believe that you should feel comfortable to go out when baby is in a napping routine. You don't need to miss the class or the party or the cuppa with friends. These things are just as important to a new parent as getting enough kip. They are life. And so is a good cup of coffee!

The reason we don't recommend doing naps on the go for all your baby's daytime sleeps is that motion and constant unfamiliar sounds, smells (and folk poking their heads into the pram or buggy) stop baby from going into a truly deep sleep. So, while they can sleep on the go, it will not be as solid and restful as a nap at home.

The best way to deal with naps when you're out and about is to try to recreate the same sleep associations you have at home (see p. 64). Use white noise, their comforter, a safe cover to block daylight – whatever is easy and practical to take with you. (This is also why having a routine will work for you, not against you when you want to go out – because baby will already be in the habit of sleeping at a particular time.)

Try a nap out of your comfort zone, whether that's out and about or at home (if you usually nap on the go). It doesn't mean it will happen but trying is like ripping off a sticking plaster. If it doesn't work out, don't worry. You will be able to make it up by bringing the next nap or bedtime earlier to compensate for an overtired baby.

Golden On-the-go Tips

- Always try to settle baby in their pram or buggy at their usual sleep time.
- Use the same (practical) sleep associations as at home – white noise, comforter, etc. (see p. 64).
- If your baby normally goes straight down for a nap at home, don't think you have to rock them to sleep when out. Keep it the same as at home, with as little fuss as possible.
- Make sure your baby can lie as flat as possible – a bassinet for small babies and a reclining buggy for those over 6 months.

- Try to make the buggy as 'dark' as possible; breathable shades can help to block out light. Just like at home, reducing external distractions will help kiddo take a longer nap.
- Your baby is likely to sleep less soundly out and about than at home, as they will be distracted by external stimuli. This is just something to be aware of as they may be cranky or unsettled when they wake, and you might need to make their next nap or bedtime earlier to compensate.
- Mix it up: if you've had several days of napping out and about, try to have a few at home to allow baby to get back into their routine. We go by a 4:3 ratio, where at least four days a week you stick to the routine, then the other three can be disrupted without causing too much overtiredness – but aim for them not to be consecutive. (Sometimes this is unavoidable if you have trips away.)
- If your baby falls asleep and it's unplanned, aim to interrupt it before 10 minutes, so they don't fall into a deep sleep and it doesn't impact nap time.

Finally, don't worry! Not every day will go to plan, and you will get back on track the next day.

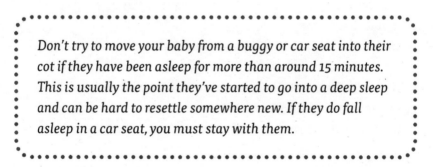

Don't try to move your baby from a buggy or car seat into their cot if they have been asleep for more than around 15 minutes. This is usually the point they've started to go into a deep sleep and can be hard to resettle somewhere new. If they do fall asleep in a car seat, you must stay with them.

Night Sleep on the Go

If you're feeling really adventurous, you might want to go out at night, too. We promise you can do that and still have a baby who sleeps. Night pram or buggy sleeps are particularly useful when you go on holiday or have a special event or dinner to go to. We recommend approaching these in the same way you would an out-and-about day nap but follow your bedtime routine before sleep.

The key things to include in your bedtime routine are getting baby's nappy changed and, if you can, popping them into pyjamas or a sleepsuit.

Give them a good feed and wind, then put them in a familiar swaddle or sleeping bag (you can get travel sleeping bags that work with harnesses in buggies or car seats). Then put them into their pram, buggy or car seat and use their usual sleep associations (see p. 64) to start their overnight sleep.

> *There are some children who really struggle to sleep well out and about. That doesn't mean you shouldn't try it. You absolutely should. Just keep your expectations low and you never know – you might be surprised!*

SURVIVAL:

If you have only ever napped on the go or only at home, carry on doing this until you feel you have established a nap routine.

MOVING FORWARDS:

Try a nap out and about, and if it doesn't happen how you expect it to, feel confident in bringing the next nap or bedtime earlier to avoid overtiredness.

Drop Naps Without Losing Sleep

Crib Notes

- Look for signs that your baby might be ready to drop a nap – like refusing or not settling at naps or bedtime, naps becoming later and early waking.

- It's ok to drop a nap and it doesn't work. Just go back and try again when ready.

- Nap transitions: from four to three naps (around 4 months), three to two (around 6 months), two to one (12 months+).

- Prevent baby from becoming overtired by bringing the next nap or bedtime earlier.

- If baby is struggling to drop a nap, use quiet time (reading a book, gentle sensory play) to help them through it.

You're happily in a routine. You finally get stuff done when baby naps. You feel like you might be nailing this parenting malarkey. Then bam! They drop a nap and you feel like you're losing more than a bit of sleep.

There are usually clear signs when baby is ready to drop a nap, often age-related, but not always. Here are some to look out for:

- Waking early in the morning (and not resettling)
- Reluctance to go for a nap
- Waking early from naps or not linking sleep cycles together
- Settling and sleeping well at one nap and not another
- One nap getting gradually later and later
- Two naps becoming one (isn't there a Spice Girls song about that?) – so a morning nap gets so late in the day that an afternoon nap becomes impossible
- Reluctance to go to bed at night

Nap Transitions

We talk about dropping a nap, like you simply chuck it on the floor and shove it under the bed with the forgotten Lego pieces. But it's often not that straightforward. It can take a while to notice the signs that baby is ready (see above); and even once you know, it can take a few weeks for baby to lose the nap entirely. There might be a few false starts along the way, with more naps on some days than others.

One of the reasons it's important to keep an eye on signs for readiness is that too much or too little day sleep can really affect night-time. It's a delicate balance.

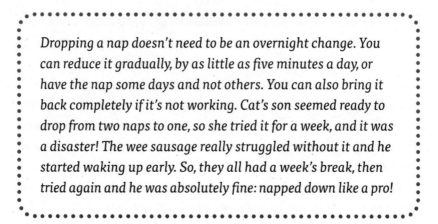

Dropping a nap doesn't need to be an overnight change. You can reduce it gradually, by as little as five minutes a day, or have the nap some days and not others. You can also bring it back completely if it's not working. Cat's son seemed ready to drop from two naps to one, so she tried it for a week, and it was a disaster! The wee sausage really struggled without it and he started waking up early. So, they all had a week's break, then tried again and he was absolutely fine: napped down like a pro!

We recommend baby going to sleep in their cot or safe sleeping space at home for all naps when they are going through a transition, as this is where they will have the most sound and restorative sleep.

And remember The Sleep Mums' Rule of Three: you should start to see changes in three to five days, so give it time before you start worrying that it isn't working.

From four to three naps (around 4 months)

This transition often happens without you even noticing as your baby's sleep needs gradually become less during the day. You will often struggle to fit in that fourth nap, whether because you are too busy doing things, they have extended the time of their other naps or they simply won't settle for it.

With this transition, you will usually see a pattern develop of one shorter nap in the morning, a longer afternoon one and a short late-afternoon one. However, there are no hard-and-fast rules – sometimes babies will settle and sleep for longer in the morning. You can choose.

From three to two naps (around 6 months)

The third nap is important in the early days, as it helps power baby through until bedtime when they are small. But at this age, we recommend this disco nap is kept on the fly – either on the go or somewhere busy that stops baby going into a deep and solid sleep – and usually less than 20 minutes. It can also be a lovely chance for a cuddle. As long as baby is having two other naps, with one over 45 minutes, this one is usually the easiest to drop.

The biggest signs that baby is ready to transition from three naps to two are their age (around 6 months), struggling to settle at bedtime and early-morning waking.

135

You can drop this nap without a major transition period, although you may find you need to bring bedtime forwards a little for a few nights as baby gets used to not having it.

If your baby struggles without the nap, you can gradually shorten it, waking them after 10 minutes, until you feel they're ready to drop it entirely.

From two to one nap (12 months+)

Dropping from two naps to one is harder, and it can take a long time for your baby to adjust. There's also a bigger variation in age for dropping it – from as early as 12 months to closer to 18 months, so look for signs rather than dates on the calendar. The most obvious are not settling during one of the naps, difficulty settling at bedtime, multiple night wakings and, again, early-morning waking (without resettling).

Transitioning to one long sleep after lunch can take time. The gentlest way to do it is to reduce the morning nap, taking it down to just 20 minutes. Then, bring lunchtime earlier and make sure they start their long sleep earlier (usually around midday). Aim for the new, longer single nap to be around two to two and a half hours, giving them enough energy to make it through to bedtime. Like the first nap drop, you may need to bring bedtime forwards if baby is getting overtired in the afternoon.

Once they are coping without the morning nap, you can gradually push lunch and afternoon nap time a little later (in 10-minute increments) towards 12.30/1pm, which usually fits in better with family life.

Your baby will continue to have one nap a day until they (or you) are ready for them to drop it.

SURVIVAL:

If you think baby is ready to drop a nap, try reducing it gradually, starting with as little as five minutes, and see if it makes a difference.

MOVING FORWARDS:

Feel confident to drop baby's nap if they are ready and use The Sleep Mums' 30-minute buffer, if required, to bring their next sleep a little earlier to prevent overtiredness.

Understand Regressions

You will no doubt have heard parents whispering about the 4-month Sleep Regression in reverential tones. There are millions of articles, blogs and guides to getting through it; everyone, including our mums, has an opinion on them. But, dear reader, we're going to blow your mind: the 4-month Sleep Regression does not exist.

We feel quite strongly about talking about this because a lot of parents get the fear as they approach 4 months (16 weeks),

138

feeling certain they're going to go back in time to the newborn days. This worry alone can impact sleep. It also means that the slightest disruption to sleep gets blamed on a regression.

People also talk about a 6-month regression, a 10-month one, a 12-month one, an any-time-my-baby-doesn't-sleep one.

You may also have heard them called sleep progressions. This is more factually correct, but it can make parents feel like they should be celebrating them. And you're unlikely to feel like cracking open the party poppers!

Regressions are often made to sound like something that happens to a baby and parents just have to bleary eyed accept it. That is not the case. We believe that by being aware of your baby's development and making sure their changing needs are met, it doesn't have to be something awful.

The Regression–Progression Question

Between 4 and 6 months, your baby's sleep changes. They move from short sleep cycles with a range of only two sleep phases to a more adult one. So, why does this mean they wake up more? Isn't a longer sleep cycle a good thing?

One reason is those pesky extra phases of sleep. Your baby starts going into a lighter phase of sleep between cycles – a phase that they previously didn't have. This means they might think it's time to get up or they are more easily disturbed; they are much more aware of their environment than they were as a newborn.

A second reason is that as your baby heads towards the half-year mark, their nutrition and sleep needs begin to change.

There are developmental shifts in their minds and bodies, they start moving more and their physical movements become smoother. All this working out and working things out means they often become hungrier and need more sleep. That's why some call it a progression – as baby is growing up.

Another reason is that because your baby is more aware now, they become harder to settle and because the parent or caregiver is more exhausted – four to five months of sleep deprivation will do that to a person – they feel less able to cope with it.

Turning Back the Clock

The sleep changes at 4 months can hit parents hard. Months of disturbed sleep can take their toll and if, as is often the case, baby has been sleeping better for the month or so before their sleep gets upended, you can find yourself wishing you could turn back the clock.

This extremely emotional side of developmental shifts doesn't get enough airtime. Your baby might be graduating in terms of sleep, but you might not be ready for them to grow up so quickly. They may need more from you to sleep better, which can be demanding, and you might find yourself longing for the newborn days.

You may feel it is too exhausting to do anything different right now but being aware of these shifts and your baby's needs will help you think about putting a plan in place. If you're not ready to make any changes yet, you don't have to. As long as your baby's needs are being met.

The 4-month Sleep Hump

You'll see that while a regression might not exist, there is definitely something going on. Your baby is reaching big developmental and physical milestones, and so are you. The changes at 4 months tend to be bigger – or at least they are most talked about when it comes to sleep disturbance because they are a perfect storm of development.

That's why we call it the 4-month sleep hump. It's something you might need to work through, but it is passable, even when sleep-deprived.

The hurdle will be bigger for some than it is for others. Some babies sail through milestones without it ever affecting their sleep, while for others it can cause a bigger impact. It will also be different for your baby at different stages.

What About the Others?

The so-called 6-month sleep regression is usually an extension of the changes that occur around 4 months. It may happen later for some babies or it may build up, and it is only when things get worse that parents realise something has changed.

People talk about 10- and 12-month sleep regressions, too. These usually occur because of the huge physical leaps babies take – first crawling and then starting to walk. And whenever a baby goes through a developmental shift their sleep can be affected.

Getting Over the Hump

When you are ready, make a plan to support your baby through the hump. Your plan might include adding top-up feeds during the day and more in the way of settling, both overnight and during their naps, to help them through the lighter phases of sleep.

Hungry Monster

As well as sleep, during times of development, your baby may need more milk (or food, once they are weaned) to give them energy. In our routines, you will see that between 4 and 6 months we include the option of top-up feeds. These set the foundations for mealtimes once baby is weaned but can also help them through the hump. They give them the extra nutrition they need to extend their longer daytime nap and give you more confidence to settle them at night, knowing they have had extra feeds in the day. They also give your baby comfort when they may be feeling unsettled – because growing up is scary (for everyone!).

Some babies can go off their feeds during developmental changes. A baby who had been settled during feeds can become fussy or push the bottle away if bottle-feeding. Continue to offer milk at the times in the routine, even if they appear not to want it. You may need to offer it and then take a break before coming back to it once they have calmed down.

Make Use of The Day

Sleep, or a lack of it, is what people mostly talk about during developmental changes. But the time your baby is awake is just as significant.

Give them plenty of opportunities during the day to practise any skills they may be learning. This will help them to process them in the day (and less likely to practise them at night!). For example, at 4 months, rolling is often the big one. At 6 months, it could be sitting up, at 10 months, walking or crawling (and at 384 months, it might be getting your own baby to sleep!). Our babies' brains are working overtime to make sense of their new skills, and this can mean they have trouble switching off when they sleep.

Baby 2.0

Often in your baby's first year you can feel like you have this parenting thing down. Then you pop them down for a nap and it feels like they wake up in version 2.0 – in less time than it took for you to do a load of laundry.

Routines are useful because they help take some of the guess-work out of your baby's needs and, hopefully, give you the confidence and space to be able to read them better. Babies go through big changes in their first year and their needs change a lot. Our routines are age-based, but listen to what your baby is telling you, too; they will show and tell you when things need to change.

So, if you suddenly find you are having very disrupted nights or days, it's a good idea to look at their routine. Are they grump-ier or hungrier? Are they waking soon after you put them down (within an hour or so) regularly through the night? Or are they waking early?

These are all signs (often ones that people talk about with regressions) that indicate that something isn't working with their routine. It may be that they need to move on to the next one early, or they need a bit of time to adjust to a new one. Sometimes it might be a few days or even a week or two until baby settles. Remember, we include the half-hour flex in all our routines to help you adapt them when you need to (see p. 35).

Parent Skillz

When your baby is going through a developmental shift, they often need more intervention from you to help them get back to sleep. So, you need to work on your settling skills. Find something that works for you and them – and it may be different from what has previously been successful.

We recommend trying out new settling techniques at naptimes, when everyone is a little less tired. Working things out during the day acts as a rehearsal and means you are both more comfortable with any settling techniques being used at night.

SURVIVAL:
The most important thing when making any changes is that you have the energy and resolve to implement them. So, wait until you do.

MOVING FORWARDS:
Give yourself and your baby a week or two to focus on getting through the hump. Start with adding in the top-up feeds. This will give you more confidence to use settling techniques to extend their daytime naps (if needed) – and always use them before feeding overnight to gently stretch the times between night feeds.

Get Some Solid Sleep: Weaning

Crib Notes

- Start weaning when you see signs that your baby is ready (around 5–6 months); these include: interest in food, greater co-ordination and seeming less satisfied by milk.

- Baby-led or spoon-fed? There is no one right way.

- Build up to three meals a day (more quickly than you might think).

- Food can make baby more windy.

- Get ready for weaning nappies!

- Foods to avoid include: honey, cow's milk to drink (but it's fine for cooking after 6 months), shellfish, salt, runny eggs (no eggs at all before 6 months), mould-ripened cheese.

- When at home, wear an apron when starting to wean!

Weaning can feel like a bit of minefield. There's so much information out there and a lot of it is quite contradictory. But it doesn't need to be a food fight.

The guidelines are very age-driven. The current recommendation is for weaning at 6 months), but lots of parents get tied up over whether it's 24 weeks or 6 months, and whether it is 6 months to the day. We recommend looking at your baby as an individual. They will likely be ready to wean around 5–6 months, but always look for signs that they are – and make sure you are, too!

Like all things in parenthood, you need to work out what works best for you and your family weaning-wise. Some children are ready before others, as are some parents. Eating solid foods can feel like a big change for baby, and while it is exciting, it can also involve a lot of work.

Solid Signs

So, how do you know when your baby is ready for food?

Babies usually become increasingly interested in what you're eating, show more co-ordinated movements, and they might even go off their milk a little. From a sleep point of view, you might start to see early wake-ups or night wakings when they have previously been sleeping through, disrupted naps and a lack of concentration during awake times.

How to Start

This is the beginning of your baby's journey into food; it's a really big milestone, but it can be overwhelming. So, have realistic expectations – your baby is not necessarily going to open their mouth straight away; this is a new skill they need to learn, and for the first few meals, it can feel like they are using their tongue to push food away. Sometimes you might offer a spoon 10 or 20 times and still end up wearing it! But baby is practising and experiencing new tastes, so please don't be disheartened.

If you are starting before 6 months, begin by introducing one meal, building up to three a day over the course of a few weeks. If your baby is 6 months or older, you will get to three meals more quickly. Pick your day and pick your first meal; there are no hard-and-fast rules about this – just choose based on what fits with your routine and allows you not to be in a hurry. Fast food isn't great for baby!

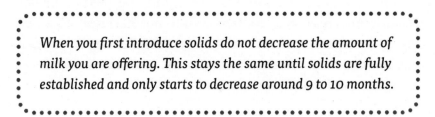

When you first introduce solids do not decrease the amount of milk you are offering. This stays the same until solids are fully established and only starts to decrease around 9 to 10 months.

There is a saying that 'Food before one is just for fun', but this isn't factually correct. We prefer our podcast guest nutritionist Charlotte Stirling-Reed's take: 'Food before one *should* be fun'. Try to make it as enjoyable an experience for you and baby as you can.

As with all things baby, there are a million gadgets and gizmos you could buy that the adverts tell you will make life easier. But here's what we think you'll need:

- Shallow, oval-shaped, soft-touch spoons
- Bowls – you can just use what you already have at home
- A silicone-spouted sippy cup – these are best for encouraging independent drinking
- Bibs – we like ones that fully cover the body and have arms
- High chair or baby bouncer; think about your space, style, how long you want it to last and cost
- Time to focus on introducing food

First Tastes

Keep it simple. Start with a sweet vegetable such as sweet potato, carrots or peas. Begin with one veg at a time, then you can mix the ones you have introduced. Veggies for breakfast are totally fine – baby doesn't know the difference and keeping their diet savoury at first is important.

Some foods may cause a rash around your baby's mouth because of a high acid content. While not harmful, it can be uncomfortable, so it is advised to avoid the following if you see it happening: citrus (oranges, tangerines, lemons), strawberries and tomatoes (including sauces).

Baby-led or Spoon-fed?

There is no one way to feed your baby, despite what some hard-core fans might have you believe. Most parents find they end up doing a little bit of both.

In the early days, if you are starting to wean any time before 6 months, always begin with spoon-fed purées. Then, when age-appropriate, you can offer finger foods. This can help you to feel more confident about the amount of solids your baby is taking.

If your baby likes to be more independent but you like them to have purées, these can also be spread on toast or rice cakes to allow them to feed themselves.

It's good for babies to feel and explore food with their hands; it's a learning experience, as well as fuel. Plus, finger foods can help to keep their hands occupied instead of hitting the spoon and covering you both in (more) food.

Water, Water Everywhere

Offer water with every meal. Babies generally don't master the art of properly drinking water until around 10 months. But even if they are only chewing and sucking slightly on the cup, they will still be getting a little on board, so it's a healthy habit to start and can help prevent constipation.

Solids Sleep

Sometimes food can have a positive effect on baby sleep. Well-fed babies with happy tummies do, generally, sleep better. Plus, some foods can actually help baby get to sleep – in particular, those that contain tryptophan (a substance which, when combined with healthy carbs, promotes better sleep).

The following foods might help with sleep:

- Oats
- Wheat
- Soya and tofu (be aware of allergies, especially if they run in the family)
- Green leafy veg, like cabbage and spinach
- Nut butters, like almonds, cashews and walnuts (be aware of allergies, especially if they run in the family)
- Bananas (mix with avocado for a hearty brekky that will set them up for a good first nap)
- Poultry (especially turkey – that's why everyone falls asleep on Christmas Day!)

However, beginning weaning is unlikely to suddenly make baby sleep through the night, if they haven't been previously. In fact, solid food can sometimes cause some sleep issues – babies' stomachs are small and not used to these lovely new tastes, so some might experience more in the way of wind, constipation and occasionally tummy aches. It's a good idea to give baby an additional massage (see p. 75) around lunchtime to help their digestive system along. It can be your trump card when it comes to sleep! Lol.

> *Gently cycling baby legs is a good way to try to move trapped wind. In Cat's house they called it pumping the poo and made up a song about it. (We may have now reached peak parent overshare!)*

Solid Poos?

Your baby's poo is going to change a lot when they start solids. Don't be scared by what you see down there – the poos can change from solid to sloshy, depending on what they've eaten, and it generally doesn't mean that there's anything wrong. You might see carrots, corn, bits of fruit. In fact, it often looks remarkably similar to how it did when it went in.

Things to look out for in poo are excessively watery consistencies after the same food, mucus in their poo and very, very bright green poo (a little green is ok). If these things persist, always talk to a healthcare professional.

Food for Life

Remember, once you start weaning your baby, you can't just stop because your days are too full and you don't have time. So please make sure you are ready before you begin.

Some days you may need to offer more finger foods or snacks if you are on the go, but still offer food at breakfast, lunch and dinner times.

Solid Gold

Once you and baby are ready to go, here are some Sleep Mums' tips for starters:

- **Begin with a mealtime when they are not too tired and not too close to a feed.** In other words, they're not starving. Look at your day and which meal works for you because there is no right or wrong; just make sure you're not in a rush. For example, breakfast around 45 minutes after their morning milk, lunch 60 minutes before their long nap and dinner approximately 2 hours before bed.

A good reason to start with a meal earlier in the day is that if the food your baby eats produces more wind than normal, they have the whole day to wiggle it out before bedtime.

- **Start with savoury purées and soft textures.** Your baby is graduating from liquid to solids, so take it gradually. A child's food should be around 85 per cent savoury and 15 per cent sweet.

There's no need to introduce sweeter foods until later. They don't know what they're missing until they've tried it.

- **But don't feel like you have to choose between purées or finger foods (if older than 6 months).** You can also do both or just one. Like most parenting decisions, it's about what works best for you and your baby.
- **It may take your baby a while to get used to the new flavours.** Don't be surprised if they reject the food or spit it out – and never take it personally! Ease them in by mixing the new food with a few teaspoons of their usual milk.
- **Meal sizes should start small.** A tablespoon in a bowl to start with is plenty. If they finish this, you can offer more. But equally, don't worry if they barely eat any. Offering food on a serve-yourself basis at the table can also really work well for older kids who don't want certain things on their plates.
- **Be a cheerleader.** One day, you will stand on the sidelines, cheering your kid on for something wonderful, like the sack race. Weaning is your first taste of being a cheerleader. Eating is a big deal, and we should make it a happy and positive experience for them by ladling on the praise. Food with a side order of 'Clever baby!' seems to go down much better.
- **Feed them until they are full.** It's important to continue to offer food to baby if they are looking for it – you will not overfeed your baby. As they adjust to solids, they will increase the amount they eat, so always be ready to offer more at each meal. This helps baby to learn – and tell you – when they are full.
- **It's quality not quantity.** One baby might be full after a few mouthfuls, while another will scoff the whole bowl. The main thing is making sure the food is good quality and baby-appropriate.
- **Your baby's appetite will vary, too.** There are a number of reasons why baby might be hungrier on some days and less

so on others (teething is often a big culprit), but as long as they have plenty of wet and dry nappies, try not to worry.

- **Always stay in the room when your baby is eating so you can monitor their chewing and swallowing.** Avoid the following choking hazards:
    - Popcorn
    - Cherries
    - Whole olives or grapes
    - Whole or chopped nuts

We recommend taking a paediatric first-aid course so you can be confident in knowing the difference between gagging and choking and how to deal with either if they occur.

- **Aim to do the 3:2.** This is not some mad diet, thankfully. We just like to use it as a structure for your baby as they head out of their first year. By the end of weaning, the aim is that your baby will be eating three meals a day and two snacks. On any given day, the actual amounts will vary but it is worth trying, to avoid the hangrys (see Glossary, p.302).

SURVIVAL:

You do not need to be up cooking purées through the night. You can, but there are fantastic shop-bought purées for baby for a reason. Your adult child will not flunk their driving test because you fed them food you didn't make yourself at 3am. Promise.

MOVING FORWARDS:

Think about increasing your baby's solid intake; if they are not yet on three meals, build up to it. And practise being their cheerleader, even if you feel frustrated about how much – or how little – they are eating. You will both get there.

Deal with Early Waking

We all miss the days of a decent lie-in but when baby is waking early doors on the regular, even 5am can feel like a bit of a luxury. Is there anything you can do to make the night-time last a bit longer?

The first thing to say is that (unfortunately) any time from 6am can be considered morning for a baby if they are going to bed around 7pm. This might not be exactly what you want to hear but some babies struggle to get past this time as they have already fulfilled their sleep needs. Anything before 6am is an early wake or a night waking. Sometimes simply calling 5.45am a night wake can help you persevere with a resettle, whereas calling it an early wake makes you feel like you should start your day.

The main reasons for early waking are poor naps, their last nap of the day being too long or too close to bedtime and too late a bedtime.

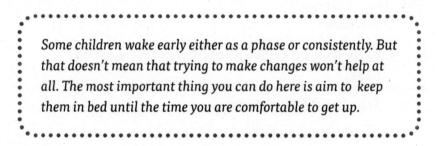

Some children wake early either as a phase or consistently. But that doesn't mean that trying to make changes won't help at all. The most important thing you can do here is aim to keep them in bed until the time you are comfortable to get up.

Over-overtiredness?

It can seem logical that the best solution to early waking is simply to put your baby to bed later. However, a big culprit when it comes to early waking is when your baby goes to bed overtired. Overtiredness increases cortisol (one of those annoying not-at-all-sleepy hormones we've talked about), and can mean your baby struggles to settle, has wakeful nights and may wake early.

Timing of naps is important, too. If baby's morning nap is too soon after waking, it can mean they use it as an extension of their night, which reinforces early waking.

And if their last nap of the day is too long or too close to bedtime, it can mean they start their night-time sleep from then, leading to early waking.

Daylight Savings

Try to get out as much as possible during daylight hours. Just like in the newborn days, early waking can create a jet-lag-like effect, so make sure you get daylight to regulate circadian rhythms. If the weather is bad or it's simply not possible, keep lights on at home during the day and ensure there is fresh air circulating, either from open windows or keeping the door ajar.

Going out for a walk at the end of the day, just before the bedtime routine, can help, too – even just for a few days to try to push their wake-up later.

Use Stop, Listen, Look (see p. 61). However, if you feel baby is very awake, it can be better to take a less-is-more approach.

Space Invaders

A number of external factors can affect early waking.

One is temperature: getting cold from kicking off blankets (that's why sleeping bags can be good) or because the heating has gone off; or sometimes the opposite, when the heating comes on or the sun hits their window.

And talking of sun, darkness can be a factor, too. We all need darkness at night to help with our circadian rhythms, and during summertime it can get lighter from the mid-point of the night. That's why we love blackout blinds throughout the year for baby's bedroom. It's also worth thinking about light leaking in from the rest of your home, especially if the door is kept open.

It's Good to be Boring

Settling techniques can work less well in the early morning because baby has already filled their tank with a decent amount of sleep. Try to avoid too much stimulation from you or an established sleep association. Basically, any settling needs to be as boring as possible; if you normally use a bum pat, now is the time to be more hands off.

The other thing is to take the small wins; if baby wakes at 5am, then only resettles until 5.15am, don't be disheartened, but do make that your benchmark for the next night, aiming to resettle until 5.20 or 5.30 the following morning. It can be a slow process, but you will get there.

Supper Club

We talk a lot about full feeds, but this can be particularly important with early waking, which can sometimes happen because baby is hungry. If you have already night-weaned your baby from milk feeds, you don't want to go back to feeding overnight. If you think hunger is why your baby is waking early, though, you can give them a pre-bath top-up feed to help fill them up. And/or if they are eating solid foods, you can give them something slow-release to sustain them until morning. Porridge, bananas or yoghurt (depending on age) are good bedtime 'snacks'.

Breaking Habits

Sometimes you can try all the above and your baby will still wake early. This can be really, really frustrating. One reason could be that your baby has simply got into the habit of waking early. That means all the other stuff – naps and food, etc. – are dictated by their early wake time, so your day is out before you even begin, and that can be a really hard thing to change. It is doable, though.

The first step is looking to see if something is out of sync in your 24 hours for baby's age and stage. The second is feeling confident using the 30-minute buffer to gradually shift things in the right direction (see p. 35).

If your baby wakes at 5am and doesn't resettle, aim to use settling techniques until as close to 6am as you can (on a 7am–7pm routine). They will look for their first nap earlier than on your typical day, but try to keep them going by using The Sleep Mums' 30-minute buffer (see p. 35) to push that first nap later. Then, when they wake up from that nap, also use the 30-minute buffer to try to push their feed or snack later. This should help you to get back on track for the day.

The Breakfast Hack

Sleep associations help to get baby to sleep but awake associations can help them to wake up at roughly the same time each morning (see 'Have a Breakfast Feed', p. 84). The aim is to try to give your baby their first feed of the day – their 'breakfast' feed – at exactly the same time every single day.

This needs to be done gradually – their hunger can take time to catch on. Gradually distract them for around 10 minutes every day from when they wake until you feed them. This will allow you to get closer to what you want their wake-up time to be. Once you are consistently feeding them at the same time every morning, this can encourage them to sleep until their hunger (their breakfast alarm) wakes them.

For example, if baby wakes at 5.30am and you would like them to wake at 7(ish) it can take several weeks of slow adjustment and perseverance. Then, once baby is able to go closer to 7am without a feed, always be consistent about feeding them at or as close to 7am as possible.

SURVIVAL:

Coping with early waking can be really tough but try to make a diary and see if you notice anything in your day that might be contributing to the early waking.

MOVING FORWARDS:

Have you tried everything? Take it slowly, fill them up at bedtime, use all the techniques in this chapter to gradually edge their awake time later and work on their wake-up routine.

Feel Comfortable Moving Your Baby into Their Own Room

Crib Notes

- **This move might be to the room next door but it can feel like another planet.**

- **The right time for this move is when you are ready. Then just go for it!**

- **Parents often find this move harder than baby.**

- **Be practical (and make a plan) . . .**

- **. . . but it's ok to be emotional, too.**

- **Let them get used to their new sleeping space; do a daytime nap there first.**

Your baby has probably been in the same room as you since they were born. Moving them can feel hard and scary. Or you may be celebrating this milestone by firmly closing their brand new blackout blinds and cracking open the champagne.

Six and Out

Official guidelines say that your baby should be in the same room as you for at least the first six months. Mostly, this is for safety, but it's also generally easier for the regular night wakes for feeds, nappy changes and settles that come with having a small baby. Plus, you can keep a watchful eye or ear on them, even when you're half asleep – which is what most of us are for those first six months!

But practically and emotionally there is no right time. You may live in a way that means you will always share space with your child, so you may choose to co-sleep or be creative with the space you have. You or your baby might be a very light or noisy sleeper, so you might choose to sleep apart to help you both get more sleep.

The other, not-so-talked-about reason why 6 months is often considered a good age to move your baby is because it slams sleeplessly into the change in their sleep patterns. We discuss this in more detail in 'Understand Regressions' (see p. 138), but around this age their sleep cycles become more adult in range. This means that they are more likely to be disturbed by parents coming to bed, snoring or passively aggressively discussing who is getting more sleep.

Practicality A-part

Your reasons for moving your baby into their own room can be very personal and differ from baby to baby. There are pros and cons to both sharing a room with your baby and moving them into a separate space. There may be consensus in a random parenting forum about what is best for your baby but, honestly, expert opinion is still out. There's also a fair amount of debate about when is the best time (and if). So, it needs to come down to what is best for you and your baby. And only you know that. But at some point you will likely decide that time is now.

You can just go ahead and do it and not look back (although you will look into their room 100 times on the first night). Or you can do it gradually, moving their cot, crib or sleep space away from you in the room, bit by bit. This can be a really gentle way to help you both get used to the idea.

Whatever you choose, here are our top tips to make the move more seamless and less sleepless once you're ready.

Safe Room

One of the biggest things about a move is you are changing your baby's familiar sleep space to an unfamiliar one. They need to feel safe and secure to feel comfortable to go to sleep and you need to know that they are, too. Spend time together in their new room, let them play in it, read stories in it and change their nappy or clothes there.

Start with at least one daytime nap to get comfy in the space, when you both will likely have more energy to deal with the change.

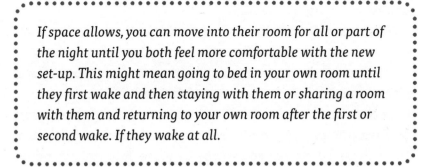

If space allows, you can move into their room for all or part of the night until you both feel more comfortable with the new set-up. This might mean going to bed in your own room until they first wake and then staying with them or sharing a room with them and returning to your own room after the first or second wake. If they wake at all.

Same, Same but Different

When you first move your baby, keep the same bedtime routine and sleep associations that they are used to (see pp. 74 and 64). Use the same sleeping bag or sheets and blankets, too, if you can. All these familiar elements let them know they are safe and nothing (much) has changed.

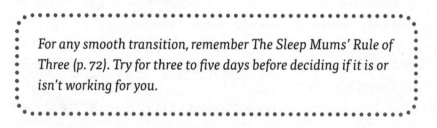

For any smooth transition, remember The Sleep Mums' Rule of Three (p. 72). Try for three to five days before deciding if it is or isn't working for you.

Most babies adjust much more easily than we as parents think they will – or than we do ourselves!

Keeping it Together

Moving baby out of your room can feel like they may as well be leaving home, getting a job and their own place. It can feel really daunting. It may also be off the back of many sleepless nights or months, so emotions are high.

Plus, this milestone can fall around the same time as many others: starting solid food, sitting up independently, blowing raspberries at you . . . It is the most grown up your baby has ever felt and this can bring out a range of different feelings.

It's ok to feel sad about it. It's a milestone, and there are very valid reasons why you might feel anxious. You might worry that they will sleep less, and you will be up more, that you will not be able to hear them or that something will happen and you're not there. These are all totally normal concerns. It can also feel a physical wrench; when you have been close to baby for their entire life (so far), being apart can bring on feelings of separation anxiety for you (probably not for your baby at this point).

As much as baby needs to be ready, you need to be ready, too. With this in mind, we recommend having a plan, as this can help with some of the bigger feelings. Knowing what is happening when and how you are going to deal with the move can make you feel more in control of it, which often helps with anxiety.

It's also worth thinking of the positives: doing adult things in your own room, like watching a movie or eating snacks in bed and not always having to tiptoe around. Why, what did you think we meant?

> *For the first few nights, you will be up and down checking on them, possibly even willing them to wake up because you miss them (if there was ever a sign parenthood makes you crazy, there it is!). At first, you may choose to keep a baby monitor on all night. However, unless your room is very far away, it's a good idea to only use this for a few nights, as it can make you feel more unsettled.*

What If the Move Makes Sleep Worse?

If you are feeling worried about the move, you may find yourself looking for perfectly plausible reasons not to do it. What if it makes sleep worse? What if I'm still feeding? What if I'm traipsing down the hall multiple times a night? What if they can't sleep without me? What if I miss their tiny pterodactyl snores?

The first thing to remember is that making a move doesn't mean it has to be for ever. Try it out; see how you both feel. You can always do a few days and think of it as a 'holiday'. And if it doesn't work, leave it for a few weeks and come back to it. But do keep trying.

The second thing to remember is not being disturbed by every snort, snore or stir – yours or theirs – often means fewer wake-ups, not more. If they're hungry or they need you, you'll know about it.

Another bonus, particularly where feeding is concerned, is that having baby in a different room can make it easier for a partner or family member to settle them.

SURVIVAL:

To cope with the move emotionally, the best plan is to move into their room with them. This can be for as long as you need to gently help you both get used to the idea.

MOVING FORWARDS:

Feel confident about the move. You will know when the time is right for you and your baby. But don't be surprised if it takes you a while to get used to the idea – even if you are ready – and think about what you can do to make it a more restful night's sleep for you, whether that is getting an early night, using a video monitor or having a bath before bed.

Know How to Wean Your Baby from Night Feeds

Crib Notes

- It's normal for babies to move away from night feeds as they get older.

- When night weaning, always look at your day first.

- Use Stop, Listen, Look (see p. 61).

- With any wake, aim to always use settling techniques first (see p. 100).

- Only do it when there are no other big changes.

- Make a plan.

People think they have a right to a say in how much sleep you or your baby needs. On the one hand, there is a badge of honour among some parents suggesting that sleep deprivation proves you're working harder as a parent, while others can make you feel you've done something wrong because your baby should have been 'sleeping through' from a few weeks. Hopefully, you know by now that we believe the only thing that really matters is what's right for you and your family.

A baby can naturally stop feeding overnight before 6 months. However, as they approach 4–6 months they may begin waking again and seem to be looking for food. For parents, feeding their baby feels like the obvious thing to do – it worked when they were younger, and they simply stopped when they were ready. However, after 6 months, a baby is less likely to stop feeding overnight without help. Look at their daytime routine to understand why they are waking and try not to reintroduce night feeds.

If your baby is 6 months or older and has never slept through the night without feeding, you may be thinking about trying to gradually shift away from night feeds. Weaning baby from feeds at night isn't a guarantee of a full night's sleep because there are loads of reasons your baby wakes up at night and hunger is only one of them. However, night weaning can be a big step towards both you and baby getting more sleep.

When to Night Wean

All babies are different. Some naturally wean from night feeds at an early stage, while others will be later (and may need a little help). On the whole, you're really looking for changes in behaviour rather than age. Here are some things to consider:

- Is your baby waking up, settling themselves, then waking up again?
- Are they feeding for less time than they have been, or taking less milk from the bottle?
- Has your baby started waking more frequently and you are feeding them at every wake?
- How are they eating and/or feeding during the day?
- Do you have a consistent routine?
- How do you as a parent feel? If baby is ready, are you?

Remember Stop, Listen, Look (see p. 61). Take a moment, take a breath, make a cup of tea or go for a pee. Then listen to your baby's cries – really listen to the sounds that they're making: are they actually just having a grumble? Could you leave them? Then look (either take a peek or use a video monitor): are they lying down? Are their eyes open? You want to have all the information you can before you go in – if you even need to go in at all.

Breastfeeding and Bottle-feeding

The main difference in night weaning if you are bottle- or breast-feeding is that it generally takes longer to make up a bottle. That means a baby who is ready to night wean may well have resettled by the time their bottle-feed has been made. It's important that if this happens, you don't give it to them. They have shown you they don't need it (at least for now). We know it feels wasteful – but it's less wasteful in the long run if they successfully drop their night feeds.

If you're breastfeeding, you'll have a physical response to stopping feeding, which can be really hard. Pump if you need to and wear someone else's T-shirt or jumper. It helps baby not to be distracted by the smell of your milk while you are settling them and, hopefully, lets everyone get back to sleep more easily. Or, if you can, ask for help resettling them while you're trying to stop feeding overnight.

Cold Turkey

It is possible to go cold turkey: simply shut up shop at the milk bar overnight and don't look back.

There are some circumstances in which stopping outright might be preferable. The first is that your baby no longer needs milk overnight. The second is that you are ready. And the third is, for example, if your baby has decided that they prefer only having milk at night and aren't taking on enough during the day – then you need to try to flip their timings around, so they're getting more milk and food on board during the day instead of looking for it at night.

In this circumstance, your baby does not know what time they are waking up and how many times they have been fed. It can, therefore, be less confusing for them to simply stop feeding overnight and use other settling techniques instead.

If you are still sharing a room with baby, it might be an idea to swap to the other side of the room or bed if this takes you a little further away from them. This extra distance can help you both get through stopping feeds at night.

Give it Some S-T-R-E-T-C-H

If you are trying to reduce night feeds but not get rid of them completely, or you would prefer a more gradual process to stopping feeding overnight, you can do it by extending the time between feeds.

The foundation of stretching out your baby's feeds comes from Stop, Listen, Look (see p. 61). As soon as you start to follow this guideline, you will see a natural stretch because there will be times when your baby will grumble and then go back to sleep.

Gentle night-weaning hacks: wear someone else's T-shirt, move your baby's sleeping space away from yours if it's still in the same room (you can do this permanently or just for the period that you are stopping feeding overnight) and be consistent – once you've made the change, stick to it.

How to gently stretch out the time between babies' feeds:

When your baby wakes up, follow Stop, Listen, Look (see p.61).

If your baby reaches a point of not settling that you feel requires assistance, go in and implement the settling techniques you have chosen (see p. 100).

Set yourself a time goal – for example, 20 or 30 minutes of settling. Then assess how you think baby sounds. If you feel they are close to sleep, persevere. You're nearly there.

If they are not going to go back to sleep, leave the room, then re-enter and feed them. This distinguishes between the settling and feeding.

Put your baby back into their cot or sleeping space aware (see 'Always Put Your Baby to Bed Aware', p. 94) and leave the room.

Follow the Stop, Listen, Look guideline again. This time, if baby doesn't settle, you don't put a time frame on implementing settling techniques (as you have recently fed them); instead, you push through until baby is fully asleep.

If you successfully settle baby without a feed, well done – it can be tough. They may wake again quickly but don't be disheartened. When you first start this process, you might need to resettle them a lot and only get an extra 15 minutes before feeding. However, the 15 minutes might become 20, or even 30 minutes the next night. And it will gradually just keep stretching and stretching and stretching.

Another tip is to set yourself little goals. You can do this right from the start. So, if your baby generally doesn't wake until 11pm or perhaps 2am, then before you start, commit to that being the first time that you will feed them. Then, if the next night they go to 12 or 3am respectively, that becomes your start time for the first feeding. And you can build from there.

You do need to be consistent to achieve this. As hard as it sounds, if you go back to feeding them earlier on the odd night, it can be harder to break the habit a second time.

Be confident in your plan, knowing you are fulfilling your baby's nutritional needs during the day by following a daytime feeding routine and making sure they have full feeds every time. And always wind baby really well after each feed (see p. 33), so that a bit of trapped wind isn't the thing keeping them up at night. Remember, discomfort from wind often looks like hunger.

SURVIVAL:

Practise stretching baby between feeds, even if it is just by small amounts.

MOVING FORWARDS:

Have a plan. Make sure you have a week where you can focus on night weaning without any other big changes going on. Set yourself goals and try to stick to them. Having a plan makes it easier on the hard days . . . and there will likely be some.

What to Do When You Have a Bad Day

Crib Notes

- Don't worry about crap naps on some days. It happens.

- If you have a bad night or nap, put baby down earlier for their next nap or bedtime.

- But don't bump all your timings too much to cover things if they go wrong.

- Break your day down into more manageable bits: morning, afternoon, evening and overnight (or even further, if all you can manage is focusing on the next hour).

- Remember The Sleep Mums' 30-minute buffer (see p. 35).

- Once baby's in a routine, don't worry about going 'off book' for a day or two.

- Tomorrow is always another day.

The key thing to remember when you have a bad day is that you can come back from it. It doesn't mean that it's over, you've failed and have to scrabble around on the floor picking up the pieces of your day like a jigsaw. One of the most common things we see when people have had a bad day is that they drop their routine completely and it ends up with a domino effect, where the next day and the next go out of whack, too.

As hard as it is, you need to try to take each day as a new one. That might sound like a parenting platitude but it's actually quite a relief when you think about it. If it all goes tits up, there's always tomorrow.

A Hard Day's Night

A bad night or day's sleep can end up making you feel like everything will go out of sync. However, that doesn't have to happen. Remember you have The Sleep Mums' 30-minute buffer either side of your routine timings to allow you to read your baby's cues and give both you and them some flexibility. You can use this buffer for every one of your timings without it affecting the routine. However, don't go over 30 minutes, as this can end up pushing any difficulties to later in the day.

A Piece of Cake?

We like to think of your day as slices of time or sections. Think of your baby's 24 hours in terms of morning, afternoon, evening and overnight.

This means that if the morning goes tits up, you can still use the afternoon and the bedtime routine to try to get things back to normal. Even if two slices, or the whole day, get messed up, you can still pull it back: tomorrow is another day. The most important piece of your day is having a start time. This is something you can always come back to after a bad day.

Give it a Flex . . .

Once baby is settled in a routine, it's generally ok to go 'off book' for a day or two without it affecting nights too much. However, if your nights become unsettled, go back to the basic structure of your routine and be more consistent again.

We know it can be hard to understand the balance between being consistent and being flexible. However, we believe being consistent most of the time affords you the ability to be flexible when you need to be.

. . . But Don't Rewind

When you have a bad day, it can be easy to slip into things you might have done when baby was younger. This might be rocking, feeding or using a particular sleep prop when you have weaned yourself and baby from it. Or feeding overnight when you have already stopped. We are not saying never do these things, as sometimes you need to – but just know that it can be harder to stop a second or even a third time.

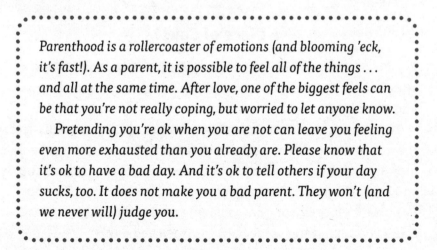

Parenthood is a rollercoaster of emotions (and blooming 'eck, it's fast!). As a parent, it is possible to feel all of the things . . . and all at the same time. After love, one of the biggest feels can be that you're not really coping, but worried to let anyone know.

Pretending you're ok when you are not can leave you feeling even more exhausted than you already are. Please know that it's ok to have a bad day. And it's ok to tell others if your day sucks, too. It does not make you a bad parent. They won't (and we never will) judge you.

Some days you will feel like you're on fire and you will nail parenting like Bob the Builder. Other days you won't. Everyone is like this; no matter what it looks like from the outside.

SURVIVAL:

If all else fails, just cuddle. It might do you both the world of good. Or, if you're feeling totally touched out, let them wriggle in a safe space (like their cot) for a little while, or ask someone to help you take a break.

MOVING FORWARDS:

Coming back from a bad day is about having the confidence to be flexible. If you have one bad day (or even a few), we want to give you the strength to know that you can keep going and remind you of The Sleep Mums' Rule of Three (see p. 72). If one part of your routine is consistently not working after five days, have the confidence to look at it and change it.

Bonus Guideline: Don't Listen to Jeff or Janet

You can gauge how much sleep matters to parents by how much they talk about it. 'Do they sleep through the night?' 'How many times are they up?' 'Why are they always awake from 1–3am?' 'Why do they wake so early?' Often, these conversations are answered by sleep-worn myths that seem to have been passed on from parent to parent for decades.

But here's why you shouldn't listen to the Jeffs and Janets of the world – those well-meaning folk at playgroups and, occasionally, parents, grandparents and mothers-in-law.

What Janet Says: A Tired Baby Will Sleep Better

Nope. Often, the reason why babies don't go to sleep is because they are overtired. The more tired they are, the more they will fight sleep. The more tired they are, the more they will fuss and cry when you put them down. The more tired they are, the less likely they are to have a good, long and restorative sleep.

So, how do you know if your baby is overtired? They will:

- fight sleep
- wake up easily
- have short naps
- be unable to link sleep cycles together by themselves
- fall asleep quickly in the car seat, buggy or while feeding

- be fussy (and get fussier as the day goes on)
- demonstrate hyperactive or excessively excited behaviour – we call it the crazy-tireds
- have frequent night wakings

If you have a good routine and are consistent about bedtimes, baby should not get tired. By keeping to a routine, they become more flexible, not less, because they are not overtired. So, they can cope better with the odd missed nap, overstimulating trip to soft play or wee bout of illness or teething.

What Jeff Says: Your Baby Will Sleep Later if You Keep Them Up Later

This never works, no matter what Jeff says. In fact, the opposite is often true. A tired baby is more likely to wake early, so putting tired kids to bed early or in time with their routine usually makes them sleep longer. We kid you not!

What Janet Says: Your Baby Will Sleep Better When . . .

. . . they're eating/crawling/3 months old/they've eaten their first birthday cake . . . People often seem to think that any of these things will change a baby's sleep patterns. In truth, the only thing that will help a baby sleep better is . . . helping a baby to sleep better!

Teaching your baby good sleep habits and getting them into a routine that ensures they are full and not overtired will help them to sleep better sooner, whatever milestone they are at.

What Jeff Says: Never Wake a Sleeping Baby

You want your baby to have their longest sleep at night. If you allow them to sleep for too long during the day, they are more likely to wake more frequently at night.

Being in a routine and waking baby at certain times to stop them from sleeping too long through the day ensures that they are the right level of tired for their next sleep (so no overtiredness), and that usually means they go down better and sleep better, both for naps and at night.

It can take a while to get your head around waking your child during the day because sometimes that nap has been difficult to achieve in the first place. However, sticking to a regular routine means baby will become more habitual in their day sleep and you can start setting your watch by them . . . ok – maybe a slightly wonky watch that kinda works sometimes!

What Jeff Says: Sleep When the Baby Sleeps

Let's be practical here. On average, a newborn will sleep up to 18 hours a day, and as amazing as that sounds, that's not going to work well for anyone.

The important thing to do when baby is sleeping is to try to look after yourself – have a shower, a proper meal, a (hot) cup of tea (rehydration is vital, especially if you are breastfeeding), watch telly and, if you can, by all means have a nap. But try not to do it in the cereal aisle.

What Janet Says: A Breastfed Baby Will Not Sleep Through the Night

If your baby is not sleeping and is breastfed, folk (like Janet) may tell you that if you give them formula, they will sleep better. This assumes two things: firstly, that the only reason baby wakes up is to be fed, and secondly, that breast milk cannot provide enough sustenance for baby to sleep through the night. It's simply not true.

As long as little one's nutritional needs are met during the day, by ensuring full and proper feeds, and they do not have any additional medical needs, there is no reason that a breastfed baby cannot sleep through the night before 6 months. If your baby is getting to sleep without props (rocking, feeding, etc.), then they will learn to sleep well and through the night, whether they are breast- or bottle-fed.

What Jeff Says: It's Just a Bit of Colic . . . They'll Grow Out of It

Colic is a very old-school term, meaning 'unexplained crying', which is pretty unhelpful. If baby seems to be very unsettled, it's unlikely to be 'unexplained'. Babies have immature digestive systems, and it can take time for their wee bodies to get used to the world. If your baby is in a lot of distress, waking frequently and seems in pain, especially during or after a feed, and you've ruled out wind or a burp, speak to a healthcare professional.

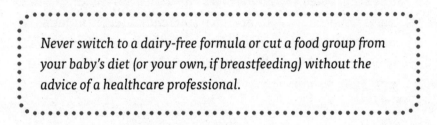

Never switch to a dairy-free formula or cut a food group from your baby's diet (or your own, if breastfeeding) without the advice of a healthcare professional.

What Janet Says: Teaching Your Baby to Sleep Will Make Them Hate You

Teaching your baby to sleep better does not have to mean leaving your baby in a dark room to cry for hours. Rest assured – helping them to settle and learn how to get themselves to sleep will not harm your baby. In fact, research has shown that there are no negative effects on parent–child bonding when teaching your child to sleep, even if it involves a few tears for you both.

Remember that by helping baby to sleep, you are helping them to grow, physically and mentally. Plus, you are giving yourself permission to sleep.

What Jeff Says: You Can't Cuddle or Sing with a Strict Bedtime Routine

Teaching your baby to settle themselves does not mean that you or your baby become robots. You don't have to stop doing the things you both love. You can always continue to do any or all those things as part of the night-time routine: consistency is the key.

Creating positive sleep associations is important – so if singing, cuddling or telling a story are part of your routine, that's a good thing. Just make sure you do it *before* your baby is asleep and you've put them to bed!

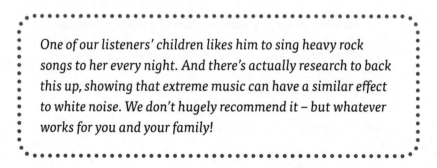

One of our listeners' children likes him to sing heavy rock songs to her every night. And there's actually research to back this up, showing that extreme music can have a similar effect to white noise. We don't hugely recommend it – but whatever works for you and your family!

What Janet Says: Putting Your Baby in a Routine is Restrictive

We believe the opposite is true. Being in a routine means that baby will be well rested and less likely to be overtired, so you can actually do more. Plus, it's more likely to be fun if you don't have a cranky baby.

Our routines are flexible and, as you've learned, hackable. You can organise your day and your baby's feeds and naps around the things you want/need to do (classes, playgroups, a sibling or school runs) without them getting tired or hungry.

What Jeff Says: Your Baby Only Wakes Because They are Hungry

This is a myth that is easy to fall into bed with because even if baby isn't hungry, they will likely take a feed and possibly fall asleep afterwards. Just not for very long.

So, you get into a cycle: baby wakes up, you feed them and they go back to sleep for a while. However, they have also now learned to expect food when they wake, so they ask for it, which means you think they are hungry when they wake up. Every. Single. Time.

If you know you are giving your baby full and proper feeds during the day, you are following a routine that is age-based and they are happy and otherwise thriving with no medical issues, you should feel confident in knowing your baby is not always hungry when they wake and it is ok to settle them without feeding first.

What Janet Says: You Can't Share a Room and Teach Baby to Settle

You can sleep in the same room as your baby during sleep settling. Being close to them might even make you sleep easier, knowing they are safe.

What Jeff Says: My Child is Just a Bad Sleeper

All babies sleep 'badly' (from an adult perspective) at the beginning, for loads of reasons: they need to be fed and cuddled often, they have much more active sleep than we do and their sleep cycles have yet to mature. However, in the majority of cases, babies (and children) are not *just* bad sleepers – they simply have habits that are preventing them from sleeping better.

> *Establishing a routine, meeting your baby's needs for food and sleep during the day and having the confidence to know what settles them will help your baby to become a better sleeper, whatever their personality.*

What Janet Says: Change Will Make You MORE tired

You're exhausted. You're hanging on by a thread. You feel like changing what you do or how you do it will push you over the edge. It's easier to keep the status quo. You're all getting a little sleep, and you simply cannot cope with it getting worse before it gets better. So, just leave things as they are, thank you very much.

That's how parents get stuck in bad sleeping arrangements for months and even years. Not because they don't know how to change, but because the thought of it seems too much. Simply too tired to get more sleep.

Change is scary and can be tiring but you're here, so you may feel you need to do something different. It might be tough for a few days, but it will get better soon and, most likely, within a few weeks.

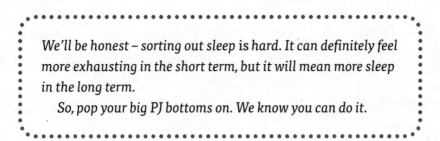

We'll be honest – sorting out sleep is hard. It can definitely feel more exhausting in the short term, but it will mean more sleep in the long term.

So, pop your big PJ bottoms on. We know you can do it.

Part III

The Sleep Mums' Routines

The basis of our routines is that they are foundations; they take some of the guess work out of your baby's needs because you are meeting them consistently. And each routine builds on the one before, so you don't need to learn a whole new one with every change.

You do not have to follow our routines from birth. Whenever you pick up this book, just jump to the age-appropriate routine for your baby.

If a routine is working for you, there are no hard rules about moving on to the next one on the exact day your baby moves up in age. Sometimes they will be ready to move on before, and sometimes after. Just keep an eye on what your baby is telling you.

Nevertheless, it's good to be aware of what the next routine looks like, so if your baby starts to become more unsettled or their sleep or feeds appear to change, you can be ready to move on. Then, take a few days for you both to get used to it. Make sure you have time – between three and five days – to focus on the changes and be as consistent as possible (see The Sleep Mums' Rule of Three, p. 72).

In our routines from 5 months we give you the option to choose a longer morning or lunchtime nap. This is because we want to give you the maximum flexibility to work our routines around your lifestyle. However, once you have decided which routine – longer morning or lunch nap – works for you and your baby it is important to be consistent.

0–2 Weeks

Crib Notes

- **It's ok to cry.**
- **Try to keep talking.**
- **Try to accept help.**
- **Keep a feeds, pee and poo diary.**

You

Congratulations – you're a parent! At first, you will be making it up as you go along. Your baby will be sorting out their likes, wants and needs, and you will be desperately trying to work out exactly what those are. You are both rookies in unknown territory.

You may be euphoric and full of life; you may also be a puddle of tears on the floor. Crying at this stage is perfectly acceptable – we have both been there and sobbed our hearts out – and the baby blues are very common (see p. 13). Please try to keep talking, read our 'No Rules for Feelings' chapter (see p. 12) and seek help if you are worried.

It is important to accept help. It can come in many forms, and while people will almost always offer to have the baby, it's ok to say no and ask them to do the washing, hoovering, cooking – or whatever you need – instead. Looking after you is looking after the baby.

Food

You will have had ideas of how you would like to feed, whether that was breast, bottle or combination. The route you take may work from the beginning, but not always.

Breastfeeding is hard. It can hurt and takes time to establish. It's a new skill to learn for you and baby, even if you have breast-fed before. Every baby is different. Trying to get the latch and position right for you both can be tough. Go easy on yourself and make the most of any support you have.

Bottle-feeding is hard, too, and can take time to establish. Like breastfeeding, it's a new skill to learn for you and baby, even if you have bottle-fed before. It requires organisation and the right equipment – suitable bottles and a way to sterilise – and patience for you both to feel comfortable going with the flow.

Plus, your baby is going to pee and poo a lot. You can expect 8–10 bowel movements in 24 hours. They will also feed regularly, roughly every two hours. You may become quite obsessed with how much baby eats, poos and pees, so we recommend keeping a simple diary to refer back and see if any patterns emerge.

Naps

Don't worry about them getting too much or too little sleep at this stage. Some babies will nap all the time; others won't.

Play

Play at this stage is more about cuddles and sleep. Skin-to-skin is the dance party of entertainment for your baby.

Your question

Q. I'm a first-time mum and I've just had a baby and he seems really sleepy. After everything you've said about baby sleep, is it possible for a newborn to sleep *too* much?

A. Some babies need a bit more sleep to recover from birth, as do their parents. You should be looking for plenty of wet and dirty nappies and still feeding regularly. If you feel that your baby is excessively sleepy or starts sleeping more than usual after the first few days, then they should be checked out by a healthcare professional.

You'll find more of your questions in our Troubleshooting Guide, p. 278.

0–2-weeks Routine

Remember, this is the Spring Break of parenting. Anything goes. The routines will get more detailed as your baby grows but for now, you are just getting to know each other.

As well as reading the 'No-rules Rule' guideline (see p. 12), here are some things that you might want to think about in the first two weeks:

- A baby needs to be fed every two to two-and-a-half hours.
- We recommend waking them to feed every three hours to feed overnight, unless you've been told otherwise.
- Wind always and for ever (see p. 33).
- Make sure you can get their tiny fingers safely out of a sleeve!
- Cuddles.
- Hearing your voice.
- Sleep – for both of you.

Growth spurt alert! *Your baby will have regular growth spurts in the first six weeks. The first is usually at about 10 days old. During these growth spurts, they may look for more milk and be a bit more unsettled. Some babies sleep less; others more. Generally, a spurt lasts 24–72 hours before things return to normal. You might have a tough few days and only notice afterwards that it was probably a growth spurt.*

2–6 Weeks

Crib Notes

- **Get to know your baby.**
- **Enjoy the cuddles . . .**
- **. . . but don't worry if you feel touched out and you need to take a break.**
- **Keep it simple.**

You

We've spoken about those first two weeks – the flooring exhaustion and the overwhelming emotions. It's intense. Often, in the early days, your body is still going on adrenaline. It helps get you through, but as the weeks creep by, tiredness can begin to set in.

If you want to stay in all day, that's ok. It can feel like you need to be back out and about doing things, even when baby is still brand new, but in some cultures, mother and baby don't leave the house for 40 days or more.

Remember, you and your baby are still getting to know each other. It's the honeymoon phase (with less sleeping and champagne). The idea in these early weeks is to lay the foundations of a routine, so you can start to be a little more aware of timings and how things might fall into place when you're ready.

The key point is to try to enjoy your baby. Snuggle them, smell them, smile at them and play with them. Sleep will come. We promise.

Some things to think about in the first six weeks:

- Space feeds by two to two-and-a-half hours.
- Make sure baby isn't overtired and that they are well fed and freshly changed before putting them in their cot, Moses basket or safe space for naps and sleep.
- Help baby to wind down, using the same techniques each time – these are your positive sleep associations (see p. 64). Change their nappy, put the lights on low, swaddle, give them a cuddle and use white noise (see p. 25).
- If they don't settle, don't worry. Have a cuddle, then try again. If they don't settle at all, get baby up, reset and/or give a top-up feed and try again when you're both ready.
- They're not robots. Like us, babies can feel extra hungry one day and not so much the next.

Food

It's a good idea to start baby's routine in the morning to help them begin to work out the difference between night and day. This would typically be between 6 and 9am. The most important thing after their morning wake-up and first feed is to make sure they take their next milk feed two to two-and-a-half hours after. Then every two to two-and-a-half hours until the end of the day.

They can often start to stretch to three hours between feeds overnight. Plus, you can still expect 8–10 bowel movements in 24 hours from your pooper trouper.

Naps

At this stage, baby will be awake for a maximum of 60–90 minutes (including feeding, winding and nappy-changing times).

Your little squish is still small, so don't put pressure on yourself; if you want to stay in your jammies and go back to bed when baby takes their naps, never feel bad about it. Everything else can wait.

Play

Nappy changes are as wild as playtime gets – seeing your facial expressions (at what's inside!) is enough stimulation for them at this age.

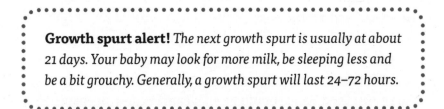

Growth spurt alert! *The next growth spurt is usually at about 21 days. Your baby may look for more milk, be sleeping less and be a bit grouchy. Generally, a growth spurt will last 24–72 hours.*

Your Question

Q. My baby is amazing at sleeping . . . on me, but an absolute nightmare anywhere else. They simply don't sleep. Is there anything I can do?

A. The first things to try are putting your baby in a swaddle and turning on white noise. Start small – take it one nap at a time – and be consistent. Use all the settling techniques you need to help them settle in their safe sleep space (see p. 100) and then gradually, over a few days (and it might be a tough few days), they will start to get the hang of sleeping somewhere other than on you.

You'll find more of your questions in our Troubleshooting Guide (see p. 278).

2–6-weeks Routine

You and your baby are just getting to know each other, so this is more of a guide than a routine. The last part of your day could look something like this:

- **4.30pm: feed** This feed will be two to three hours after their previous one.
- **5/5.15pm: nap** Baby may take a short nap following this feed, depending on how they have slept during the day.
- **5.45pm: bath time or short massage (see p. 75)** Baby doesn't need a bath every night – every three to four nights or even less is fine. If you are bathing them, it should be kept relatively short – 10 minutes tops – as they can get cold and then struggle to sleep.
- **6.15pm: feed** Baby should be all clean, in their sleepsuit or pyjamas and swaddle or sleeping bag. Do this feed in the room they are due to sleep in and only use dim lights to try to keep everything calm and quiet. Once they have finished feeding, wind them really well (see p. 33). This is essential because even a little bit of trapped wind can cause baby to wake and be in discomfort through the night. Once you are

satisfied they are full, and all their wind is up, put baby into bed for the night (probably between 6.30 and 7pm, depending on how long they have fed).

- **Overnight** Feed on demand (but approximately every three hours). Only change their nappy at night if they have done a poo. They need to get used to a wet nappy at night so they don't wake up whenever it's wet.

No two days are likely to be the same at this stage, and if these timings don't fit with your day, it's ok to adapt them to work for you and your family.

6–12 Weeks

Crib Notes

- **Don't compare where you or your baby are at with others.**

- **Feeds and naps become more defined (but don't worry if they don't).**

- **Continue to swaddle and use positive sleep associations (see p.64).**

- **Your baby may start to do longer stretches at night.**

You

You have survived the first six weeks. Sometimes people think this is the magic number and that it will all fall into place and get easier from here. For some it does and for others it doesn't, so please don't focus on a particular age when you think you should be managing. It's ok to be where you are; try not to compare yourself to others.

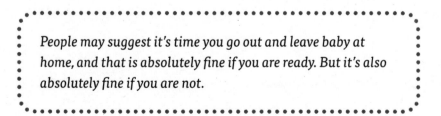

People may suggest it's time you go out and leave baby at home, and that is absolutely fine if you are ready. But it's also absolutely fine if you are not.

Newborns are hard. Getting a baby to fall asleep and stay asleep can be hard. However, the more hoops you jump through, often the harder it can become.

We have been that parent (well, Cat has) who walks the streets desperately trying to get their baby to sleep. Many get to the point where they will do anything to get even five minutes' rest. That's where stories of driving across the country (been there), buying a ludicrously expensive vibrating seat (done that) and jiggling baby until they go to sleep (got the milk-stained T-shirt) come from. But the best advice we can give you is to keep it simple.

Growth spurt alert! *The last of the first big growth spurts is around 6 weeks. Your baby will feed more regularly and often be more unsettled. They may sleep more or less. It should pass after 24–72 hours. It can be hard work, but try to go with their needs during these times.*

Food

Baby will still be feeding very regularly; you do not want to be going longer than three hours during the day. However, if they are gaining weight, feeding is going well and there are no medical concerns, you can start to leave them a little longer overnight if they are asleep. Offering full feeds and winding well are still essential.

Naps

Your baby will still need a lot of naps in the day, but these will become more defined as they reach 12 weeks. If you are swaddling your baby, do it for all naps and overnight. If you use a Moses basket or similar, use the same routine for naps as you do at night. Ensure the room is dark and the temperature remains consistent.

Always follow safe-sleeping guidelines. Put baby to sleep on their back, make sure their feet are at the foot of their cot or Moses basket and there are no loose covers or blankets near by.

Play

You will be getting short bursts of awake time now involving more interaction with your baby. At this age and stage, it can be a fine line between positive play and overstimulation. Keep an eye on them – turning away, not wanting to look you in the face and nuzzling into you are often signs they are ready to call it a day with play.

Here are some examples of simple play for your baby:

- Eye-to-eye contact
- Black-and-white toys and books
- Gentle singing
- Soft, quiet, sensory toys
- Reading (can be anything, not just baby books)

Your baby will likely only be able to cope with around 5–10 minutes of play. You may see glimmers of smiles, starting with the eyes and moving to their mouth. Don't worry if you don't, though. All babies develop at their own pace.

Baby development is a bit like popcorn (stick with us here) . . . Kernels that are cooked in the same pan at exactly the same temperature all pop at different times. Your baby will pop when they are ready.

Your Question

Q. I have tried everything, but my baby just won't sleep in her Moses basket. How can I think about a routine if she won't sleep on her own?

A. This is probably the top question we are asked by parents in the first 12 weeks. It's really important to help your baby settle in their sleep space, but you need to be ready to commit to doing so. It may take a little time, so a routine and consistency are key. When you decide you are ready, put your baby in their basket and use settling techniques to help them go to sleep. It can feel hard at first, especially if you're used to them sleeping on you. However, if you're satisfied your baby has had enough food and is not overtired, you should have the confidence to settle them knowing that their needs have been met.

You'll find more of your questions in our Troubleshooting Guide (see p. 278).

Make sure their room is a good temperature; not too hot and not too cold. Aim for as dark as possible and use a white-noise app or toy to save you shushing them all night (see p. 25).

6–12-week Routine

This routine is a recommendation. Timings can be adjusted to suit your needs and lifestyle. The key things at this stage are to have a beginning and an end to your day and evenly spaced feeds. The later naps aren't set in stone because they will depend on the times of feeds and how long they last. As with all our routines, they have a flexibility buffer of 30 minutes either side of the timings, so you can read your baby.

- **7am: awake** When you are ready, choose a time that suits your lifestyle to start your day. You do not need to rush this; just start to gradually introduce a time that works for you. These timings are based on 7am–7pm, but even with a routine your baby's active time can vary.

  Offer a milk feed and then a nappy change. Feeding at this stage plus winding can take over an hour.
- **8.30am: nap** Baby will only be managing about 90 minutes of awake time just now. But don't let anyone tell you they're boring! Put them to bed for their first nap in their Moses basket or your chosen place for them to sleep. We recommend swaddling for every nap and overnight sleep at this stage. You can also use a sleep sound, such as white noise. The exact time of this nap will adjust, depending on the time of their wake-up and first feed.
- **10am: milk feed** Baby may start looking for this two and a half hours after their first feed.
- **11.30am: nap** Roughly time for baby to nap again. Again, they will start looking for sleep around 90 minutes after they woke up. Now is a good time to go out for a walk or lunch if you feel up to it.

- **1pm: milk feed** This is the longest you would want baby to have gone without milk at this stage, so offer it before three hours if they are looking for it.
- **2.30pm: nap** This is a good time for you to have a sleep as well, if you feel that you can, or at least a lie-down. This nap will usually be a bit shorter, around 40–60 minutes.
- **4pm: milk feed** Again, this is the longest baby will go without a feed, so offer it earlier if they are looking for it. Try to make this feed a really good one, ahead of the T/witching Hour(s) (see p. 91) and to help stave off late-night cluster feeding (see p. 44).
- **4.30pm: nap** Let baby get snuggled in, if you can and want to, and let them sleep on you. This can be a good chance for you to relax and enjoy each other (but it can be harder to do if you have other children). By 12 weeks, make sure this nap is no longer than 40 minutes.
- **5.45pm: bath time or a short massage (see p. 75)** Use a thermometer to ensure the bath is no hotter than 37°C. Keep a close eye on this and take baby out as the temperature cools. A bath shouldn't be too long, so your baby doesn't get cold or overtired.
- **6.15/30pm: milk feed** Time for more milk. Take your time with this feed and make sure baby has had enough and is well winded (see p. 33) before you put them to bed.
- **Overnight** Baby will be feeding on demand, but start thinking about when they are looking for food. Aim to make each feed overnight a minimum of three hours from the previous one and do not wake them for a feed, unless there is a medical reason to do so or they require milk feeds to be timed to gain weight.

3 Months

You

You may now be starting to age your baby in months (or you may end up with a 936-week-old leaving home). Either way, your baby is a proper wee human now. They will be smiling (those first cheesers can make all the sleepless nights fade away – well . . . almost) and becoming more vocal.

Sometimes, you'll need to do what you need to do to make it through the day. And that's always ok. You may have been doing that up until now: baby only sleeping on you, your partner or a boob or, perhaps, popping your little one in a carrier or pushing them in a pram until they fall asleep. At some point, though, you'll want to find consistency in a routine, and look for other ways to get your baby to sleep.

Often, the more tired you are, the less you want to put elements of a routine in place. However, for some, having no structure at all can be more exhausting, as no one knows what's happening next. So, instead of telling yourself that baby will only sleep here or there and only at these times, think about making changes and following a routine.

A nap routine becomes increasingly important because good naps can mean more consistent night sleep and, in turn, that can also mean better naps. Use our settling techniques to make sure babies have full and proper naps (see p. 100).

Food

You will still be offering milk five/six times a day.

Naps

Your little one now needs four naps: usually one not long after they first get up, another towards the end of the morning, one mid-afternoon and a shorter one later on.

Play

Your baby may be now showing signs of rolling over, from their tummy to their back. Be aware of this and always think about safety. You may also want to gradually wean them from their swaddle if you have been using one.

A few ideas for play with your baby at this age include: bubbles, balloons attached to their feet, sensory mats, signing and reading, soft rattles.

Settling

To ensure baby is getting enough sleep across the 24-hour period you may have to do some resettling. We always recommend gentle techniques. By trying some settling at this point you are giving them the opportunity to stretch their natural sleep pattern, but don't put pressure on yourself or baby. Settling to sleep can be through lifting, white noise, shushing sound or rain noises, rubbing tummy, rolling baby on to their side and patting their bottom before rolling them on to their back again. And/or baby may still need a feed to settle.

Your Question

Q. My baby won't take a bottle. Not from me or anyone!

A. Some recommend introducing a bottle early on and doing it regularly to keep it familiar, but don't despair if you haven't. With a bit of perseverance, you will get there, even when you start later. Some advice for bottle-feeding your baby: think about the teat and find a shape that doesn't leave gaps at the side of baby's mouth, as this will let air sneak in and can cause more in the way of wind. (See 'How to Help Baby Take a Bottle', p. 52.)

If your baby is still small, get cuddled up close, rock gently and wiggle the bottle as you put the teat in their mouth. This pours some of the milk into their mouth, which should help to get the suckling action going. Some babies prefer to be cradled in a more upright position when feeding.

If baby is trying to breastfeed from you when you are trying to give them a bottle, try lying them on a pillow facing away from you on their side and put the bottle in at a right angle. It means they will not smell your own milk as much.

Babies often seem to like the strangest of positions for feeding and it's very individual. (You can bet that the one that gets baby going at first will be something weird that involves you getting pins and needles!)

You'll find more of your questions in our Troubleshooting Guide (see p. 278).

3-months Routine

- **7am: awake** If baby is still waking overnight, make this wake-up different by opening the curtains, turning on the lights and speaking in a clear, enthusiastic voice. Change your baby's nappy and then offer milk, breast or bottle.
- **8.30am: nap** Sometime between now and 9am it will be time for baby to nap. This can be done at home, in a pram or, if required, the car (e.g. if an older sibling needs to be taken to school or you need to be out somewhere). We advise you to wake them from this nap after 60 minutes, so they will still have their second nap.
- **10am: milk feed** After this feed is a good window for some active play, a walk or a class.
- **11.30am: nap** Again, baby will start looking for sleep around 90 minutes after they woke up. Now is a good time to go out for a walk or lunch if you feel up to it.
- **1pm: milk feed** This is the longest you would want baby to have gone without milk at this stage, so offer it before three hours if they are looking for it.
- **2.30pm: nap** Baby will be showing tired signs again, and it's a good time for you to rest as well, as often the night feeds can make you dip in energy towards the end of the day.

- **4pm: milk feed** Again, this is the longest baby will go without a feed, so offer it earlier if they are looking for it. Try to make this a really good feed ahead of the T/witching Hour(s) (see p. 90) and to help stave off late-night cluster feeding (see p. 44).
- **4.30pm: nap** Let baby get snuggled in, if you can and want to, and let them sleep on you. This can be a good chance for you to relax and enjoy each other (but harder to do if you have other children). By 4 months, make sure this nap is no longer than 40 minutes.
- **5pm: milk feed** This feed is only if you feel they need a small energy boost to see them through this time of the day when they can be a little grouchy – also known as the T/witching Hour(s) (see p. 90) – and they may not have it every day.
- **5.45/6pm: bath time or short massage (see p. 75)** The bath should be kept relatively short (10–15 minutes tops), as baby can get cold and then struggle to sleep.
- **6.15/30pm: milk feed** This should be done in the dimly lit bedroom. If you are using a sleeping bag, put baby in it before starting. If using a noise device, start to play it when you are doing their final wind. Winding after this feed is perhaps the most important of all, as you do not want baby waking after a short burst of sleep feeling uncomfortable. When you are satisfied baby has finished feeding and is sufficiently winded, it's time for bed. Follow the same routine every night, e.g. kiss, cuddle, into bed, 'night night', lights off and then leave the room.

    Once you have left the room, take a minute to listen and give baby a chance to settle. If you feel baby does not sound like they will settle, return and use settling techniques (see p. 100).

- **Overnight** Make sure any night feeds are done in a dimly lit room and try to keep stimulation to a minimum. Only change a nappy if baby has done a poo. You can give baby a chance to settle by themselves when they wake and if they don't, use your settling techniques (see p. 100).

4 Months

Crib Notes

- Baby is becoming more alert.

- And growing – possibly out of swaddles and Moses baskets.

- Baby may be hungrier and looking for more feeds.

- Teething and drooling may have kicked up a gear.

Baby

Your baby is 4 months old and developing faster than you can imagine. It's an exciting time, but it can come with big changes and challenges. You may have heard of the 4-month sleep regression (see 'Understand Regressions', p. 138). Again, we want to reassure you that it does not need to be a problem if you are a step ahead with meeting your baby's needs. We cannot emphasise enough the importance of a consistent start and end time to your day.

There are a number of changes for your baby around 4 months. Firstly, you will start to notice them being more alert and involved, as they seem much more present in the world. They will play games with you and enjoy picking things up, feeling textures and being much more engaged in your facial expressions.

They may be ready to move out of their Moses basket and to transition out of their swaddle.

You

There might be changes for you, too. Sometimes, the pressures of late nights, early mornings, the impact of pregnancy and birth and the hugeness of this life change can take a toll on how you feel you're coping. If so, try not to be hard on yourself – you're doing a great job and you will get there. And it goes without saying, we've got your back.

The key to a good routine is keeping it. So, while you may feel exhausted trying to stick to it, this is often when having one can matter even more. If something isn't working, don't be afraid to tweak it. Our routines are flexible and, as you hopefully know, can be hacked to allow you to work out what's best for you.

Food

Milk is very much the main part of your baby's diet and will continue to be for quite some time. Your baby will now be taking between four and six milk feeds in 24 hours. It is still important to wind during and after every feed.

Naps

Baby will now have three clear naps, the middle one usually being the longest. However, if you would like to try a longer morning nap – either because it suits your lifestyle or baby prefers it – we will show you how to plan your day in our routines (see p. 213). When you are going through a routine transition, we recommend main naps are done at home for at least a week.

Prepare the room in the same way that you would for bedtime and use the same routine.

Play

Baby is now more active and many, but not all, will roll over around this age. To encourage these developmental milestones, you can help them with arm placement and gently rocking them from side to side. Tummy time is still important to strengthen back, neck and arm muscles, which helps with the skill of rolling and sitting up. You can also support baby between your legs or with cushions to begin the transition to sitting. A few ideas for play with your baby at this age include: peekaboo, reading stories, rattles and musical instruments, water mats, sensory blankets.

Settling

To ensure baby is getting enough sleep across the 24-hour period, you may have to do some resettling. We always recommend gentle settling techniques – lifting, white noise, shushing sound or rain noises, maybe a feed, tummy rubbing, rolling baby on to their side and patting their bottom before rolling them on to their back again.

Your Question

Q. My baby was sleeping so well day and night and now they have stopped? Why?

A. The shift between the 3- and 4-month routine can be one of the hardest to navigate, because your baby's sleep needs change a lot around this stage. Their sleep cycles also start to mature somewhere between 4 and 6 months, lengthening out to be more like an adult's. This development is a great thing, but it might not feel like it because this cycle milestone can also be the start of them struggling to link their sleep together. The key is having the confidence to resettle if they wake after 40 minutes.

As a result, it's a good idea to set some time aside to really focus on this routine change. Firstly, if your baby hasn't had a bedtime routine until now, introduce one and make sure you use the same sleep associations for bed and nap time. Be aware of the reduction of naps (from four to three) and the spacing of their feeds, usually stretching out to three hours if they have previously been shorter.

> *Remember The Sleep Mums' Rule of Three: it will generally take at least three days to instil new nap habits, so stick with it. You'll get there. Promise.*

You'll find more of your questions in our Troubleshooting Guide (see p. 278).

4-months Routines

Our babies are not robots. The timings below can be adjusted across the day to suit your routine. And remember, you have half an hour each side to accommodate flexibility, e.g. if baby was to wake up at 6.30 rather than 7am or sleep until 7.30am, that still works with the same routine.

The following routines are suitable for a baby who is steadily gaining weight and has no medical or feeding issues.

Longer Lunch Nap Routine

- **7am: awake** If baby has woken during the night, make this wake-up different by opening the curtains, turning on the lights and speaking in a clear, enthusiastic voice. Change baby's nappy and then offer milk, breast or bottle.
- **8.30am: first nap** Sometime between now and 9am is time for baby to nap. This can be done at home, in a pram or, if required, the car (e.g. if an older sibling needs to be taken to school or you need to be out somewhere). We advise you to wake them after 60 minutes, so they will still have their second nap.
- **10am: milk feed** After this feed is a good window for some active play, a walk or a class.
- **11.15am: small feed** You can offer a small top-up feed at this time if your baby woke and fed early after the first nap to help settle them down for a long nap.
- **11.30am: nap** Your baby will likely be showing tired signs; they can now sleep for up to two-and-a-half hours. If they wake before 90 minutes, try using settling techniques to extend the nap (see p. 100). It's fine to use a noise aid for the duration of this nap. Timings will change as baby gets older, so by 5 months they will be going for this nap at 12.30pm.
- **1.30pm: milk feed** This could be as early as 1pm or as late as 2pm. Timing will adjust later as your baby's naps change. Now is the perfect time to get outside for a long walk, meet friends or go to a class. If possible, allow baby a chance to have a play.
- **3.30pm: nap** Your baby will likely be ready for another nap around about now. This can be up to 60 minutes.
- **4/4.30pm: milk feed** This is when we recommend stacking feeds with a planned set of cluster feeds (see p. 44). The idea is to give them an energy boost to see

them through this part of the day when they can be a little grouchy – also known as the T/witching Hour(s) (see p. 90). A short play, where possible naked, in warm, soft, fluffy towels is a good idea ahead of bath time. Babies find it more comfortable being on their tummies when naked and often attempt to roll, so it is a good thing to practise. The room should be kept warm with no draughts.

- **5.45/6pm: bath time** The bath should be kept relatively short (10–15 minutes maximum), as baby can get cold and then struggle to sleep.
- **6.15/6.30pm: milk feed** This should be done in the dimly lit room. If you are using a swaddle or sleeping bag, put baby in it first. If using a noise device, start to play it when you are doing their final wind. Winding after this feed is perhaps the most important of all, as you do not want baby waking after a short burst of sleep feeling uncomfortable.

  When you are satisfied baby has finished their milk and is sufficiently winded, it's time for bed. Follow the same routine every night – e.g. kiss, cuddle, into bed, 'night night', lights off and then leave the room.

  Once you have left the room, take a minute to listen and give baby a chance to settle. If you feel they don't sound like they will settle, return and implement settling techniques (see p. 100).
- **Overnight** If you are feeding overnight, try to keep stimulation to a minimum, only changing a nappy if baby has done a poo. Ideally, you want to give them a chance to settle by themselves when they wake and then try to assist with settling. If they do not settle, and you are still offering milk overnight, this is when you would feed. Making these small changes and not always feeding straight away is a gentle method of pushing baby's timings out and allowing their natural sleep pattern.

Longer Morning Nap Routine

- **7am: awake** If baby is still waking overnight, make this wake-up different by opening the curtains, turning on the lights and speaking in a clear, enthusiastic voice. Change baby's nappy and then offer milk, breast or bottle.
- **8.30am: small feed** You can offer a small top-up to help baby settle for a longer nap.
- **9am: nap** This can be done at home, in a pram or, if required, the car (e.g. if an older sibling needs to be taken to school or you need to be out somewhere). It can be up to two-and-a-half hours.
- **11.30am: milk feed.** After this feed is a good window for some active play, a walk or a class.
- **1pm: nap** Baby will be showing tired signs. This nap should be 60 minutes. If their morning nap was on the move, it's good to try to get this one at home.
- **3pm: milk feed** Now is the perfect time to get outside for a long walk, meet friends or go to a class. If possible, allow baby a chance to have a play.
- **4/4.30pm: nap** Your baby will likely be ready for another nap around now. It can be up to 60 minutes.
- **5pm: milk feed.** This does not need to be a big feed as baby will be having another around 6/6.30pm. It just gives them a wee energy boost to see them through this period of the day when they can be a little grouchy – also known as the T/witching Hour(s) (see p. 90).

A short play, where possible naked, in warm, soft, fluffy towels is a good idea ahead of bath time; babies find it more comfortable being on their tummies when naked and often attempt to roll, so it is a good thing to practise. The room should be kept warm with no draughts.

- **5.45/6pm: bath time** The bath should be kept relatively short (10–15 minutes maximum), as baby can get cold and then struggle to sleep.
- **6.15/6.30pm: milk feed** This should be done in the dimly lit bedroom. If you are using a swaddle or a sleeping bag, put baby in it before starting. If using a noise device, start to play it when you are doing their final wind. Winding after this feed is perhaps the most important of all, as you don't want baby waking after a short burst of sleep feeling uncomfortable.

  When you are satisfied baby has finished feeding and is sufficiently winded, it's time for bed. Follow the same routine every night – e.g. kiss, cuddle, into bed, 'night night', lights off and then leave the room.

  Once you have left the room, take a minute to listen and give baby a chance to settle. If you feel they don't sound like they will settle, return and implement settling techniques (see p. 100).
- **Overnight** If you are feeding overnight, try to keep stimulation to a minimum, only changing a nappy if baby has done a poo. Ideally, you want baby to have a chance to settle by themselves when they wake and then try to assist with settling. If they do not settle, and you are still offering milk overnight, this is when you would feed. These small changes and not always feeding straight away are a gentle method of pushing baby's timings out and allowing their natural sleep pattern.

5 Months

Crib Notes

- **Baby may be seeming hungrier.**

- **They might be ready to drop the third nap.**

- **They may start (lovingly) blowing raspberries in your face!**

- **You may need to rely on hands-on settling techniques more.**

Baby

Five months! How did that happen? You may feel like time is flying, even if the days (and nights) sometimes feel long. As you head towards baby's half-birthday, it can seem like there are numerous changes, and possibly challenges, on the way. The biggest change during the next month is that your baby may be becoming more interested in food and may seem hungrier.

Developmentally, your baby will be increasingly interested in their surroundings. They might be starting to show the family skills, like rolling, sitting and interacting with you.

You

Parenting, like sleep, is always a work in progress. Five months in and you might start to be feeling confident in some things. You know your baby better than anyone else. You may feel knee deep in your new normal (and laundry) and you're ok with that. You might have been using Stop, Listen, Look (see p. 61), so you feel like you are beginning to understand your baby's cries better. You may know how to settle them and how they like to be held.

Or you might not feel like that at all – because 5 months is the in-betweeners of your first year of parenthood. You might feel daunted by the big changes around the corner. As a result, you can feel like you're not actually ready to move on from having a very small baby. Plus, your baby might not be quite ready for solid food but seem hungrier and more demanding than they have been.

So never feel like it's not ok to admit that you don't know something, are struggling or need some help.

Food

Milk is very much still the main part of your baby's diet and will continue to be for quite a long time. You will see more and more signs that your baby is ready to start solids.

Whether you wait until the 6-month (24-week) point or introduce solids beforehand, weaning your baby is a key part of their development. When you are ready to wean, you'll notice that the top-up feeds we started to introduce in the last routine will be when baby has their lunch and dinner. These become increasingly important until solids are introduced, as baby will likely be needing the extra nutrition. The introduction of solids does not affect their main milk-feed timings at all.

Here are some signs that baby might be getting ready to join the kids' table:

- Chewing and sucking on hands and toys
- An increase in demand for breast/formula milk
- Waking at night after sleeping better
- Waking earlier in the morning
- Being interested in what goes in and out of your mouth
- Starting to grab at food and drink

Naps

Your baby will still be having three clear naps a day, the middle one usually being the longest. Some babies will start to show signs of dropping the third nap, particularly as you head towards 6 months (see 'Drop Naps Without Losing Sleep', p. 133).

When going through a routine transition we recommend that main naps are at home for at least a week, where possible, preparing the room in the same way that you would for bedtime and using the same routine.

Play

Tummy time and sitting practice are still very important. In addition, you will see that your baby is copying more and more of your facial expressions, as well as possibly mimicking sounds, such as blowing raspberries.

A few ideas for play at this age include: mirror play, reading stories, musical instruments, singing, building blocks (cardboard or rubber), sensory baskets.

Settling

To ensure baby is getting enough sleep across the 24-hour period, you may have to do some resettling. We always recommend gentle settling techniques – white noise, shushing or rain noises, rubbing or patting their tummy, The Sleep Mums' Shoogle (see Glossary, p. 304), rolling baby on to their side and patting their bottom before rolling them on to their back again for sleep (if they are confidently rolling from front to back and back to front, they may naturally roll around their sleeping space or cot at night).

Your Question

Q. **All my friends' babies are sleeping through the night, but I feel like my daughter is getting up more than ever. Can you help?**

A. Your baby is developing at a rate of knots now and becoming more and more active. As a result, they are burning more fuel and so may need more to keep them going. If you or your baby are not quite ready to wean on to solids, you can juggle your day routine to include two or three extra top-up milk feeds. This will give you more confidence at night to try some settling techniques and establish longer stretches of settled sleep. Only do this when you are ready, though, as it can take time and commitment.

You'll find more of your questions in our Troubleshooting Guide (see p. 278).

5-months Routines

Our babies are not robots and the timings below can be adjusted across the day to suit your routine. And remember, you have half an hour each side to accommodate flexibility – so, if baby wakes up at 6.30am rather than 7am or sleeps until 7.30, that still works with the same routine.

The following routines are suitable for a baby who is steadily gaining weight and has no medical or feeding issues.

Longer Lunch Nap Routine

- **7am: awake** If your baby is waking overnight, make this wake-up different by opening the curtains, turning on the lights and speaking in a clear, enthusiastic voice.

  Change your baby's nappy and then offer milk, breast or bottle.
- **[7.45am: breakfast** This is when you would do breakfast once you introduce solid food.]
- **8.30am: nap** Sometime between now and 9am it's time for your baby to nap. This can be done at home, in a pram or, if required, the car (e.g. if an older sibling needs to be taken to school or you need to be out somewhere).

  We advise you to wake your baby after 60 minutes, so they will still have their second nap.
- **10am: milk feed** After this feed is a good window for some active play, a walk or a class.
- **11.30am: small feed or lunch** You can offer a small top-up time to help your baby settle down for a longer nap. If you have weaned baby, offer solids now with a drink of water.
- **12/12.30pm: nap** Your baby will be showing tired signs. Ideally, you want this nap to be at home as it is longer and the one baby will keep for longest. They can now sleep for up to two-and-a-half hours. If they wake before 90 minutes, implement settling techniques as recommended (see p. 100). It is fine to use a noise aid for the duration of this nap.

- **3pm: milk feed** Your baby will likely look for this feed as soon as they wake up from their last nap.

    Now is the perfect time to get outside for a long walk, meet friends or go to a class. If possible, allow your baby a chance to have a play.
- **4.30pm: nap** Your baby may still need a short nap at this time of day, but no longer than 20 minutes. Some days they may not take this nap, and that is fine.
- **5pm: feed and/or dinner time** Offer your baby a feed. Once you have weaned, you can also offer a small milk feed as well as solids.

    A short play, where possible naked, in warm, soft, fluffy towels is a good idea ahead of bath time; babies find it more comfortable being on their tummies when naked and often attempt to roll, so it is a good thing to practise. The room should be kept warm with no draughts.
- **6pm: bath time** The bath should be kept relatively short (10–15 minutes maximum), as your baby can get cold and then struggle to sleep.
- **6.30: milk feed** This should be done in the dimly lit bedroom. If you are using a sleeping bag, put your baby in it first. If using a noise device, start to play it when you are doing their final wind. Winding after this feed is perhaps the most important of all, as you do not want baby waking after a short burst of sleep feeling uncomfortable.

    When you are satisfied your baby has finished feeding and is sufficiently winded, it's time for bed. Follow the same routine every night – e.g. kiss, cuddle, into bed, 'night night', lights off and then leave the room.

    Once you have left the room, take a minute to listen and give your baby a chance to settle. If you feel baby does not sound like they will settle, return and implement settling techniques (see p. 100).

- **Overnight** If you are feeding overnight, try to keep stimulation to a minimum, only changing a nappy if your baby has done a poo. Ideally, you want them to have a chance to settle by themselves when they wake and then try to assist with settling. If they do not settle, and you are still offering milk overnight, this is when you would feed. These small changes and not feeding straight away are a gentle method of pushing baby's timings out and allowing their natural sleep pattern.

Longer Morning Nap Routine

- **7am: awake** If your baby is waking overnight, make this wake-up different by opening the curtains, turning on the lights and speaking in a clear, enthusiastic voice. Change baby's nappy and then offer milk, breast or bottle.
- [**7.45am: breakfast** This is when you would do breakfast once you introduce solid food.]
- **8.30am: small feed** You can still offer a small top-up feed to help baby settle down for a longer nap.
- **9am: nap** This can be done at home, in a pram or, if required, the car (e.g. if an older sibling needs to be taken to school or you need to be out somewhere). This nap can be up to two-and-a-half hours.
- **11.30am: milk feed or lunch** Offer a milk feed. If you have weaned your baby, offer solids now with a drink of water.

  After this feed is a good window for some active play, a walk or a class.
- **1pm: nap** Your baby will be showing tired signs. This nap should be 60 minutes; if their morning nap was on the move, try to get this one in at home.

- **2.30pm: milk feed** Now is the perfect time to get outside for a long walk, meet friends or go to a class. If possible, allow baby a chance to have a play.
- **4.30pm: nap** Your baby may still need a short nap at this time of day, but no longer than 20 minutes. Some days they may not take this nap, and that's fine.
- **5pm: feed and/or dinner** Offer your baby a feed at this time. Once you have weaned, you can also offer a small milk feed as well as solids.

  A short play, where possible naked in warm, soft, fluffy towels is a good idea ahead of bath time; babies find it more comfortable being on their tummies when naked and often attempt to roll, so it is a good thing to practise. The room should be kept warm with no draughts.
- **6pm: bath time** The bath should be kept relatively short (10–15 minutes maximum), as your baby can get cold and then struggle to sleep.
- **6.30pm: milk feed** This should be done in the dimly lit bedroom. If you are using a sleeping bag, put your baby in it first. If using a noise device, start to play it when you are doing their final wind. Winding after this feed is perhaps the most important of all, as you do not want baby waking after a short burst of sleep feeling uncomfortable.

  When you are satisfied your baby has finished their milk and is sufficiently winded, it's time for bed. Follow the same routine every night – e.g. kiss, cuddle, into bed, 'night night', lights off, then leave the room.

  Once you have left the room, take a minute to listen and give baby a chance to settle. If you feel they do not sound like they'll settle, return and implement settling techniques (see p. 100).
- **Overnight** If you are feeding overnight, try to keep stimulation to a minimum, only changing a nappy if your

baby has done a poo. Ideally, you want them to have a chance to settle by themselves when they wake and then try to assist with settling.

If they do not settle, and you are still offering milk overnight, this is when you would feed. These small changes and not feeding straight away are a gentle method of pushing baby's timings out and allowing their natural sleep pattern.

6 Months

Crib Notes

- **Focus on food: three meals, two snacks and four to five milk feeds.**

- **Your baby's sleep cycles will begin to lengthen.**

- **Watch for power naps becoming danger naps (see p. 126).**

- **You may need to switch up your settling techniques as baby becomes more active.**

Baby

Six months can be a really exciting age because there are so many firsts: starting solids (if they haven't already), sitting up by themselves and beginning to crawl. Over the next few months, your baby will move more, and sleep is a big part of helping them get going. They will also get tired from moving more, so should increasingly sleep more soundly. Especially as their sleep cycles begin to lengthen.

If your baby hasn't already, it's time to drop their third nap and try to make sure the first two day naps are good ones. By 6 months, a nap too late in the afternoon can really affect your baby's bedtime and lead to early waking. If your baby is up at

4am or 5am consistently, it's not because they want to meditate and watch the sunrise. Make sure they aren't napping too late in the day and taking their 12 hours of night-time sleep from their last nap.

Starting baby on solids is a huge part of their growth and development. If they are waking frequently at night, check the amount of solids they are having during the day. You want to make sure they are fulfilling their nutritional needs in daylight hours so they're not waking up hungry at night.

You

You've made it to 6 months. Give each other – or yourself, if baby isn't playing – a high five! You now have a superactive, wriggly, giggly baby. But don't worry if you're not feeling the enthusiasm – the months of pure exhaustion might be taking their toll.

Weaning is, literally, a bit like Marmite. Some parents love it – sharing the starters of baby's first foods (at 5pm nothing tastes as good as baby's leftovers). But it can also be stressful – you might feel under pressure to wean in a particular way and to be batch cooking, and your little one might not be impressed by the whole idea. They might not want to eat anything you make, and you may be worrying about how much they're having; or they might *only* seem to want to eat food that you have made, meaning late-night cooking sessions for you. They might not want to eat anything off a spoon or won't touch finger food; or they might only seem to want to eat things off the floor!

We want to reassure you – take each day as it comes and try not to be disheartened. Keep trying. How your baby eats now is not an indication of how they will eat as a toddler, a teenager or, honestly, even next week.

Food

Now you should definitely introduce solids, if you haven't already. You will be aiming for three meals, two snacks, plus four to five milk feeds a day. Your baby can now eat lots of lovely food and have some finger foods – and you may wish you had a dog to clear up the mess!

You may find your baby takes a little while to give up any top-up feeds you introduced prior to starting solids. They may not have one for a few days, and then seem to ask for it again. Follow your baby's cues and feel confident to give them what you think they need.

Naps

Your baby needs two clear naps – usually a shorter one in the morning and a longer one after lunch, but there are no hard-and-fast rules here. Some babies prefer a longer morning nap; you can find our routines for both below.

Where possible, we recommend that when going through a routine transition, naps are at home for at least a week. Prepare the room as you would for bedtime and use the same routine to get them to sleep.

Play

Your baby may now be confidently rolling over, but don't worry if they aren't – just keep practising. Your little one will be copying you even more now, so try clapping, waving and, of course, high fiving!

A few ideas for play with your baby at this age include: bubbles, stacking toys, sensory mats and bottles, handprint painting, action songs and rhymes.

Settling

To ensure baby is getting enough sleep across the 24-hour period you may have to do some resettling: white noise, shushing or rain noises, rubbing tummy, rolling baby on to their side and patting their bottom before rolling them on to their back again. Baby should still go to sleep on their back but if they are confident rolling, they may move in the night.

You may need to switch settling techniques as your baby grows and becomes more active. They may also prefer a slightly firmer pat or rub than previously.

Your Question

Q. **My baby boy is ready to be in a room of his own. It's just next door, but we can't work out how to move him into it – it feels like moving him to another planet!**

A. Transition slowly. Start by moving their sleep space away from you. You can move it little by little. If you have an en suite, you can even use that as a temporary measure for both of you to get used to the increased distance. When you're ready to make the move, get a baby monitor to give you confidence. It will feel really strange at first, and you might have a few sleepless nights as you find yourself checking on them regularly. (See 'Feel Comfortable Moving Your Baby into Their Own Room', p. 161, for more.)

You'll find more of your questions in our Troubleshooting Guide (see p. 278).

6-months Routines

The timings below can be adjusted across the day to suit your routine. Remember, you have half an hour each side to accommodate flexibility; so, if baby was to wake up at 6.30am rather than 7am or sleep until 7.30am, that still works with the same routine.

The following routines are suitable for a baby who is steadily gaining weight and has no medical or feeding issues.

Longer Lunch Nap Routine

- **7am: awake** If your baby is waking overnight, make this wake-up different by opening the curtains, turning on the lights and speaking in a clear, enthusiastic voice.

  Change your baby's nappy and then offer milk, breast or bottle.
- **7.45am: breakfast** Your baby needs to get used to savoury tastes, so offering vegetables is totally acceptable.
- **9am: nap** This can be done at home, in a pram or, if required, the car (e.g. if an older sibling needs to be taken to school or you need to be out somewhere) and should last a maximum of 30 minutes. We advise waking them after this time, to allow for their milk and a second nap.
- **10am: milk feed** You can now offer a small snack after this milk.

  After this feed is a good window for some active play, a walk or a class.
- **11.45am: lunch** You may need to play around with the timings of this meal when you are starting out with weaning. It can be as early as 11am to ensure baby isn't too tired for this exciting new experience.
- **12.30pm: nap** Your baby will be showing tired signs. Ideally, you want this longer nap to be at home as it is the

one they will keep for longer. Baby can now sleep for up to two-and-a-half hours. If they wake before 90 minutes, implement settling techniques, as recommended (see p. 100). It is fine to use a noise aid for the duration of this nap.

- **3pm: milk feed** You can offer a small snack after this milk. Now is the perfect time to get outside for a long walk, meet friends or go to a class. If possible, allow baby a chance to have a play.
- **4.45pm: dinner** Make this a good, filling meal, offering options (and plenty of encouragement).
- **5.45/6pm: bath time** The bath should be kept relatively short (15–20 minutes maximum), as baby can get cold and then struggle to sleep. When you're ready to go to the bathroom to prepare for the bath, take the opportunity to do a bit of massage (see p. 75). The room should be warm with no draughts (you still don't need to do a bath every day; once every two/three days is fine).
- **6.30pm: milk feed** This should be done in the dimly lit bedroom. If you are using a sleeping bag, put your baby in it first. If using a noise device, start to play it when you are doing their final wind. Winding after this feed is perhaps the most important of all, as you do not want baby waking after a short burst of sleep feeling uncomfortable.

  When you are satisfied baby has finished their milk and is sufficiently winded, it's time for bed.

  Follow the same routine every night – e.g. kiss, cuddle, into bed, 'night night', lights off, then leave the room.
- **Overnight** Once you have popped baby into bed and left the room, listen to how they sound, rather than just going straight back in. Follow our Stop, Listen, Look guide (if you have a video monitor) – see p. 61. If baby looks or sounds like they are just having a grumble, leave them for a little

while to see if they settle themselves. If the grumble turns into more of a cry or you feel they are not going to settle by themselves, return to the room and use settling techniques (e.g. if they're on their back, rub their tummy or head; if they're on their front, pat their bottom). Use these techniques until baby is calm and then leave the room and follow the same guidelines again.

This process can be repeated as many times as required, or if you feel your little one is not responding to being left, stay with them until they are asleep and, over time, you can help them towards settling on their own.

Longer Morning Nap Routine

- **7am: awake** If your baby is waking overnight, make this wake-up different by opening the curtains, turning on lights and speaking in a clear, enthusiastic voice.
  Change baby's nappy, then offer milk, breast or bottle.
- **7.45: breakfast** Your baby needs to get used to savoury tastes, so offering vegetables at breakfast is acceptable.
- **9am: nap** This can be in a pram or, if required, the car (e.g. if an older sibling needs to be taken to school or you need to be somewhere), but ideally at home to ensure a sounder sleep. Aim for two to two-and-a-half hours, and if baby wakes before 90 minutes, persevere with resettling.
- **11.30am: milk feed** You can now offer a small snack after this milk. After this feed is a good window for some active play, a walk or a class.
- **1pm: lunch** You may need to play around with the timings of this meal when you are starting out with weaning. It can be as early as 12.15pm to ensure baby isn't too tired for this exciting new experience.

- **2pm: nap** Your baby will be showing tired signs. Ideally, you want this nap to be at home if the morning one was on the move. If baby has slept for under two hours, let them have 60 minutes now. If they had a good nap in the morning, 40 minutes now is enough.
- **3pm: milk feed** Milk and a small snack. Now is a perfect time to get outside for a nice long walk, meet friends or attend classes. If possible, also allow baby a chance to have a play.
- **4.45pm: dinner** Make this a good, filling meal, offering lots of options. There will now be time for a play after dinner. High-chair toys are good for this time of day, allowing you an opportunity to tidy after dinner.
- **5.45/6pm: bath time** The bath should be kept relatively short (15–20 minutes), as your baby can get too cold and then struggle to sleep. When you're ready to go through to the bathroom to prepare for the bath, take the opportunity for a bit of massage (see p. 75). The room should be warm with no draughts. (You don't need to give a bath every day; once every two to three days is fine.)
- **6.30pm: milk feed** This should be in the dimly lit bedroom. If you are using a sleeping bag, put your baby in it first. If using a noise device, start to play it when you are doing the final wind. Winding after this feed is perhaps the most important of all, as you do not want baby waking after a short burst of sleep feeling uncomfortable. When you are satisfied your baby has finished their milk and is sufficiently winded, it's time for bed. Follow the same routine every night – e.g. kiss, cuddle, into bed, 'night, night', lights off, leave the room.
- **Overnight** Once you've popped your baby into bed and left the room, you want to listen to how they sound, rather than just going straight back in. Try to follow our Stop, Listen,

Look (if you have a video monitor) – see p. 61. If baby looks or sounds like they are just having a grumble, leave them for a while to see if they settle themselves. If the grumble turns into more of a cry or you feel they are not going to settle by themselves, return to the room and use settling techniques (e.g. if they're sleeping on their back, rub their tummy or head; if on their front, pat their bottom). Do this until they're calm, then leave the room and follow the same guidelines again.

This process can be repeated as many times as required, or if you feel your little one is not responding to being left, stay with them until they are asleep and, over time, help them towards settling on their own.

7 Months

Crib Notes

- **Your baby might start to recognise their name (or nickname).**

- **Food becomes a bigger part of their day.**

- **Pop out bubbles at playtime.**

- **Think about settling techniques as they become more active.**

Baby

Your baby will be building on all the skills they have learned over the last few months, and you may be feeling like they are not such a wee baby any more. They could even be starting to recognise their own name. Unless you've mostly called them peanut, monkey or Princess Fluffychops, in which case they will be more likely to respond to that! They will now be established on solids, sitting up and interacting a lot more.

If your baby is waking frequently at night, check the amount of solid food and milk they are having during the day. You want to make sure they are fulfilling their nutritional needs in daylight hours so they're not waking up hungry at night.

You

In some ways, you might feel like you've gone back to the newborn days, trying to fit in all the feeds and meals that your baby now needs. It is a lot. However, the intensity of it all does calm down. And rice cakes will soon become your very best friends.

You might have thought that weaning would be the last hurdle to getting a good night's sleep. If you're struggling with night-times, really think about using your settling techniques (see p. 100). Sometimes, when babies are up feeding a lot at night, they have less need to fulfil their nutritional requirements during the day. If you and your baby are ready, check out 'Know How to Wean Your Baby from Night Feeds' (p. 167) to give you an idea of how to gently shift their food focus to during the day.

Food

You will now be offering three meals and two snacks. Aim to make these meals a little lumpier and offer plenty of safe finger foods as snacks and/or alongside meals. You will still be offering milk four or five times a day.

Naps

Your baby now needs two clear naps, usually a shorter one in the morning and a longer one after lunch, but there are no rules. Some babies prefer a longer morning nap. You can find routines for both on pages 239 and 241.

Where possible, we recommend that when going through a routine transition, naps are at home for at least a week. Prepare the room as you would for bedtime and use the same routine to get them to sleep.

Play

Your kid's love affair with bubbles may start right about . . . now! Watch as their eyes follow them until they pop. Bubbles also make for cute pictures for the album. Their motor skills will be getting better, too – that rattle they were given as a baby may suddenly become their favourite toy (and your least). They will also become more aware of object permanence (when something is there and when it is not), which could be the start of them wondering where you are when you leave the room.

Ideas for play include: peekaboo, looking in the mirror, bubbles, putting toys just out of reach during tummy time, putting a toy in a box and helping them to open it to see what's inside.

Settling

You may have to do some resettling both at naps and overnight – white noise, shushing or rain noises, rubbing tummy, rolling baby on to their side and patting their bottom before rolling them on to their back again and, if baby is now sleeping on their tummy (because they can roll themselves over), you can pat them on their bottom.

Baby can now usually go to sleep on their tummy and be allowed to fall asleep in their chosen position, as long as they can roll comfortably. Always observe safe-sleeping guidelines by keeping their sleep space clear. Only have your chosen comforter in the cot with them.

You may need to switch settling techniques as your baby grows and becomes more active, moving around the bed. They may also prefer a slightly firmer pat or rub than previously.

Your Question

Q. I started weaning expecting my baby to eat everything in sight and be more content, but he isn't doing either!

A. When you start weaning it can be a slow process. You can feel like you go two mouthfuls forwards and then one bite back. Often your baby will take a spoonful of food and it comes out again immediately. So, you play the Hokey Cokey (in, out, in, out, shake it all about), until he learns the skill of taking food into his mouth and swallowing it. It can take time to get used to finger foods, too; you may offer a stick of cucumber only for him to stare at it for the whole of lunch time. Make it easy on yourself by not cooking elaborate meals at this stage. And stay calm. This is a normal transition and will pass.

You'll find more of your questions in our Troubleshooting Guide (see p. 278).

7-months Routines

The timings below can be adjusted across the day to suit your routine. And remember, you have half an hour each side for flexibility – so, if baby wakes up at 6.30am rather than 7am, or sleeps until 7.30am, that still works with the same routine.

The following routines are suitable for a baby who is steadily gaining weight and has no medical or feeding issues.

Longer Lunch Nap Routine

- **7am: awake** If your baby is waking overnight, make this wake-up different by opening the curtains, turning on the lights and speaking in a clear, enthusiastic voice.

Change your baby's nappy and then offer milk, breast or bottle.

- **7.45am: breakfast** You can now start to offer porridge, cereal or toast.
- **9am: nap** This can be at home, in a pram or, if required, the car (e.g. if an older sibling needs to be taken to school or you need to be out somewhere) and should be a maximum of 30 minutes, after which we advise you to wake them, so they will fit in their second nap.
- **10am: milk feed** You should offer a small snack after this milk. Start to monitor this feed, as you may see a slight reduction in how much they have. After this feed is a good window for some active play, a walk or a class.
- **11.45am: lunch** Make this a good, substantial meal to sustain baby through their longer nap.
- **12.30: nap** Baby will show tired signs. Ideally, you want this nap to be at home as it is the one they will keep for longer. Baby can now sleep for up to two-and-a-half hours. If they wake before 90 minutes, implement settling techniques, as recommended (see p. 100). It's fine to use a noise aid for the duration of this nap.
- **3pm: milk feed** Offer a small snack after this feed. Now is the perfect time to get outside for a long walk, meet friends or go to a class. If possible, allow baby a chance to have a play.
- **4.45pm: dinner** Make this a good, filling meal, offering options (and plenty of encouragement).
- **5.45/6pm: bath time** The bath should be kept relatively short (15–20 minutes), as your baby can get cold and then struggle to sleep. When you're ready to go to the bathroom to prepare for the bath, take the opportunity for a bit of massage (see p. 75). The room should be warm with no draughts. (You don't need to do a bath every day; once every two to three days is fine.)

- **6.30pm: milk feed** This should be in the dimly lit bedroom. If you are using a sleeping bag, put them in it first. If you're using a noise device, start it when you are doing their final winding. Winding after this feed is perhaps the most important of all – you don't want baby waking after a short burst of sleep feeling uncomfortable.

  When you are satisfied baby has finished their milk and is sufficiently winded, it's time for bed. Follow the same routine every night – e.g. kiss, cuddle, into bed, 'night night', lights off and then leave the room.

- **Overnight** Once you have popped your baby into bed and left the room, listen to how they sound, rather than just going straight back in. Try to follow Stop, Listen, Look (if you have a video monitor) – see p. 61. If baby looks or sounds like they are just having a grumble, leave them for a while to see if they settle themselves. If the grumble turns into more of a cry or you feel they're not going to settle by themselves, return to the room and use settling techniques – e.g. if they're sleeping on their back, rub their tummy or head; if they're on their front, pat their bottom. Use these techniques until baby is calm, then leave the room and follow the same guidelines again.

  This process can be repeated as many times as required; or if you feel your little one is not responding to being left, stay with them until they are asleep and, over time, you can help them towards settling on their own.

Longer Morning Nap Routine

- **7am: awake** If your baby is waking overnight, make this wake-up different by opening curtains, turning on lights and speaking in a clear, enthusiastic voice. Change baby's nappy and then offer milk, breast or bottle.

- **7.45am: breakfast** You can now start to offer porridge, cereal or toast.
- **9am: nap** This can be in a pram or, if required, the car (e.g. if an older sibling needs to be taken to school or you need to be somewhere), but ideally at home to ensure a sounder sleep. Aim for two to two-and-a-half hours, and if baby wakes before 90 minutes, persevere with resettling.
- **11.30am: milk feed** You should now offer a small snack after this milk. After this feed is a good window for some active play, a walk or a class.
- **1pm: lunch** Make this a good, substantial meal to sustain baby through the afternoon.
- **2pm: nap** Your baby will be showing tired signs. Ideally, you want this nap to be at home if the morning one was on the move. If your baby slept for under two hours earlier, let them have 60 minutes now. If they had a good nap in the morning, 40 minutes is enough.
- **3pm: milk feed** Milk and a small snack. Now is a perfect time to get outside for a walk, meet friends or attend classes. If possible, also allow baby a chance to have a play.
- **4.45pm: dinner** Make this a good, filling meal, offering lots of options. There will now be time for a play after dinner. High-chair toys are good for this time of day, allowing you an opportunity to tidy up after dinner.
- **5.45/6pm: bath time** The bath should be kept relatively short (15–20 minutes), as your baby can get too cold and then struggle to sleep. When you're ready to go through to the bathroom to prepare for the bath, take the opportunity for a bit of massage (see p. 75). The room should be warm with no draughts. (You don't need to give a bath every day; once every two to three days is fine.)
- **6.30pm: milk feed** This should be in the dimly lit bedroom. If you are using a sleeping bag, put your baby in

it first. If using a noise device, start it when you are doing the final wind. Winding after this feed is perhaps the most important of all as you don't want your baby waking after a short burst of sleep feeling uncomfortable. When you are satisfied they have finished their milk and are sufficiently winded, it's time for bed. Follow the same routine every night – e.g. kiss, cuddle, into bed, 'night, night', lights off, leave the room.

- **Overnight** Once you have popped your baby into bed and left the room, listen to how they sound, rather than just going straight back in. Try to follow Stop, Listen, Look (if you have a video monitor) – see p. 61. If baby looks or sounds like they are just having a grumble, leave them for a little while to see if they settle themselves. If the grumble turns into more of a cry or you feel they are not going to settle by themselves, return to the room and use settling techniques. So, if they're sleeping on their back, for example, rub their tummy or head; if on their front, pat their bottom. Use these techniques until baby is calm and then leave the room and follow the same guidelines again.

This process can be repeated as many times as required; or if you feel your little one is not responding to being left, stay with them until they are asleep and, over time, you can help them towards settling on their own.

8 Months

Crib Notes

- **You may have a more clingy baby now . . .**

- **. . . and a mini-me, as they try to copy you.**

- **They may be pushing boundaries.**

- **And you might find you need to start saying 'no'.**

- **Your baby may want more control at mealtimes, so finger foods are important.**

Baby

Babies of this age experience a developmental growth spurt. As a result, you may be aware of them beginning to form stronger attachments to people and things. Separation anxiety can become common around this stage. You may also notice them copying sounds you make and seeing facial expressions change. You may start to feel like you're getting an indication of their future personality, too.

There can be an increase in using sounds to get your attention, and your baby will now stop and look if you change your tone – for example, saying 'no' in a firm voice as they reach up towards your extra-large coffee cup will now be more likely to get their attention.

You

Being focused on looking after your baby for the last eight months can mean that you have run out of time or energy to look after yourself. It can be strange to make yourself a priority but looking after you is one of the best things you can do for your baby.

Sarah is notoriously bad at taking time out for herself. However, when I remind her that it's for her kids, she often finds it easier to give herself the excuse to take some. So, we have a phrase that we like to say, and we'd like you to use it whenever you're questioning whether you should do something for you. Say to yourself (in a dramatic voice): 'Do it for the children. Go on, you owe it to them!'

You might feel frustrated or overwhelmed at times, especially if you're not getting any space for yourself. It's ok to put your baby somewhere safe, like their cot, or ask someone to hold them while you go and take a deep breath in the bathroom or hide in a cupboard and have a scream. We have both done this many, many times.

Food

You will be offering three good meals a day, which will be increasing in lumpiness and texture, as well as two good snacks. Remember to be led by your baby for portion sizes; it's always better for them to finish a plate/bowl of food and then offer more. They will tell you when they are full. Giving them their own bowl and spoon with a small amount in it is a good idea, but you keep one, too, so you know how much they are actually eating.

Baby will have been having four milk feeds a day, but by around 9 months they will start to show signs of dropping one. It's usually the mid-morning one that goes first, but as with everything else – think about your baby's needs and follow their cues.

Naps

No big changes with naps. Your baby will continue to need two for quite a while. Be especially aware of the 'danger nap' around this age, though (see p. 125), as it can really impact bedtime.

Play

You will be getting a lot of interaction now: giggles, hand clapping and waving. Their favourite game will be foot chewing and grabbing things (often hair, necklaces, anything expensive and breakable). Some babies will now be crawling and even pulling themselves up to standing. Most will be confidently rolling and sitting up.

Ideas for play include: peekaboo, simple large-piece jigsaws, messy play with food, stacking toys, possibly a walker, talking, playing and reading together.

Sleep

You should now be getting more consistently settled nights. Although we talk about babies and children sleeping through, they do still progress through sleep cycles, so when they are in a light sleep cycle, they are more likely to become fully awake if the environment alters (e.g. change in temperature, room becomes lighter/darker, unexpected noise). Often, during the lighter sleep phase, baby will become wrigglier and possibly make some noise, too. The key thing is feeling confident that they are ok and don't need anything; it's just like when we roll over in the night and go back to sleep.

Your Question

Q. My teething baby has gone off their milk – what should I do?

A. If you know the pain of having toothache, you'll understand how teething feels. It's really ouchy! Babies just don't know how to tell us that. Often 'going off' their milk is a way of showing us they don't feel like themselves and that their mouths hurt. The best thing to do is give them lots of cuddles. You can try some pain relief (like paracetamol) about 20 minutes before feed, which will sometimes help them to suck more easily. Make sure to stick to your pain relief's guidelines. Don't let them chew on you or the teat of a bottle for comfort or relief – encourage them to use teething toys or even a fridge-cooled flannel instead.

> *Once baby is weaned on to solids, you can give them a cold banana or a homemade ice lolly (using your milk, a substitute milk or fruit and vegetable pouches) to help soothe sore gums.*

You'll find more of your questions in our Troubleshooting Guide (see p. 278).

8-months Routines

Our babies are not robots and you will still have some broken nights or disrupted days. And remember, you have half an hour each side for flexibility – so, if baby was to wake up at 6.30am rather than 7am or sleep until 7.30am, that still works with the same routine.

The following routines are suitable for a baby who is steadily gaining weight and has no medical or feeding issues.

Longer Afternoon Nap

- **7am: awake** Offer milk.
- **7.45am: breakfast** Porridge, cereal, pancakes, toast or an assortment of options.
- **9am: nap** This should be no longer than 30 minutes. If you are putting your baby into their bed at 9am and they are taking longer to get to sleep, push it back to 9.15 or 9.30.
- **10am: milk and a small snack** For example, rice cakes, houmous or toast.
- **11.45am: lunch** If possible, make this a good meal – e.g. spaghetti Bolognese, risotto, lasagne, fish pie, soup with bread. You want to offer lunch before your baby is too tired to ensure they are nice and full ahead of their next nap.
- **12.30: nap** Where possible, this should be at home. This is the nap that baby will drop last, so it's the longest of the day. It can be up to two-and-a-half hours. If your baby wakes before 90 minutes, try to resettle them to ensure they are getting enough sleep across the day. It's also ok to mix things up; so, if one day you are out all day, baby can sleep wherever you are – buggy, car seat or even the floor!

- **3pm: milk and a small snack** Now is a perfect time to get outside for a nice long walk, meet friends or attend classes. If possible, also allow baby a chance to have a play.
- **4.45pm: dinner** Make this a good, filling meal, offering options (and encouragement). There will now be time for a play after dinner. High-chair toys are good for this time of day, allowing you an opportunity to tidy up after dinner.
- **6pm: bath time** Using a sitting support can make bath time more fun. Don't fill the bath fully – just enough for a good splash. And don't spend too long over the bath but let them have fun.
- **6.30pm: bedtime** You want to be in your baby's room now getting ready for their last feed of the day. If you are using a sleeping bag, put baby in it first. If using a noise device, start it when you are doing the final wind. Winding after this feed is perhaps the most important of all, as you don't want baby waking after a short burst of sleep feeling uncomfortable. When you are satisfied baby has finished their milk and is sufficiently winded, it's time for bed. Follow the same routine every night – e.g. kiss, cuddle, into bed, 'night, night', lights off, leave the room.
- **Overnight** Once you have popped your baby into bed and left the room, listen to how they sound, rather than just going straight back in. Try to follow 'Stop, Listen, Look (see p. 61). If baby looks or sounds like they are just having a grumble, leave them for a little while to see if they settle themselves. If the grumble turns into more of a cry or you feel they are not going to settle by themselves, return to the room and use settling techniques (so, if they're sleeping on their back, rub their tummy or head; if they're on their front, pat their bottom). Use these techniques until baby is calm, then leave the room and follow the same guidelines again, if needed.

Longer Morning Nap

- **7am: awake** Offer milk.
- **7.45am: breakfast** Porridge, cereal, pancakes, toast or an assortment of options.
- **9am: nap** This should be two to two-and-a-half hours. If baby wakes before 90 minutes, persevere with resettling. Ideally, you want this nap at home, if possible.
- **11.30am: milk and a small snack** For example, rice cakes, houmous or toast.
- **1pm: lunch** If possible, make this a good meal – e.g. spaghetti Bolognese, risotto, lasagne, fish pie, soup with bread. You want to offer lunch before your baby is too tired to ensure they are nice and full ahead of their next nap.
- **2.30pm: nap** Your baby will be showing tired signs. Ideally, you want this nap to be at home if the morning one was on the move. Cap this nap now at 30 minutes.
- **3pm: milk and a small snack** Now is a perfect time to get outside for a nice long walk, meet friends or attend classes. If possible, also allow baby a chance to have a play.
- **4.45pm: dinner** Make this a good, filling meal, offering options (and encouragement). There will now be time for a play after dinner. High-chair toys are good for this time of day, allowing you an opportunity to tidy up after dinner.
- **6pm: bath time** Using a sitting support can make bath time more fun. Don't fill the bath fully – just enough for a good splash. And don't spend too long in the bath (around 15–20 minutes is good), but let them have fun!
- **6.30pm: bedtime** You want to be in your baby's room now getting ready for their last feed of the day. If you are using a sleeping bag, put baby in it first. If using a noise device, start it when you are doing the final wind. Winding after this feed is perhaps the most important of all, as you do not

want baby waking after a short burst of sleep feeling uncomfortable. When you are satisfied baby has finished their milk and is sufficiently winded, it's time for bed. Follow the same routine every night, e.g. kiss, cuddle, into bed, 'night, night', lights off, leave the room.

- **Overnight** Once you have popped your baby into bed and left the room, listen to how they sound rather than just going straight back in. Try to follow 'Stop, Listen, Look (see p. 61). If baby looks or sounds like they are just having a grumble, leave them for a little while to see if they settle themselves. If the grumble turns into more of a cry or you feel they are not going to settle by themselves, return to the room and use settling techniques (e.g. if they're sleeping on their back, rub their tummy or head; if they're on their back, pat their bottom). Use these techniques until baby is calm and then leave the room and follow the same guidelines again, if needed. This process can be repeated as many times as required, or if you feel your little one is not responding to being left, stay with them until they are asleep and, over time, work on helping them to settle themselves.

9 Months

Crib Notes

- **Your baby might be on the move.**

- **Solid food should be more established, so milk feeds will start to change.**

- **Sleep is, hopefully, more consistent.**

- **Beware of overtiredness, environmental changes and hunger impacting on early waking.**

Baby

You will be finding life pretty busy – keeping an eye on your roly-poly baby, possibly even chasing a crawling one. Solids are now more established and, as a result, their feeding routine will be starting to change.

Between 8 and 9 months, babies often begin to form attachments to people and things. They notice when something that was there isn't any more, which is heaps of fun when it's a jack-in-the-box; not so much when it's you. It can be particularly brutal when your gorgeous baby starts screaming whenever you leave the room. This is what is referred to as separation anxiety.

You

Separation anxiety can be particularly tough for you because it often coincides with you having a greater need for time apart. If you have yet to experience the nursery, childcare or grandparent drop-off, it can be one of the most heart-wrenching parts of baby's first year.

And that's the thing with separation anxiety. We often learn about it from a baby's perspective, but it affects you, too, the intensity depending on your own temperament, just as it does for babies.

In whatever way it shows up for you, there are ways to try to manage the feelings. Being aware of it is the first step. Worrying about your child is natural but if it is debilitating, you may need to talk to a professional. When you are away from your baby, try to keep yourself busy. Focus on the reunion and try to make it positive for both of you. Reassuring them can often be the first step to reassuring yourself.

Food

Continue offering three good meals a day, increasing lumpiness and texture, as well as two good snacks. Be led by your baby for portion sizes; it's always better for them to finish a plate/bowl of food and then offer more if they seem hungry or ask for it. They will tell you when they are full. Giving them their own bowl and spoon with a small amount in it is a good idea, but you should keep one too, so you know how much they are eating.

It's likely they will now start to show signs of dropping one of their milk feeds. It is usually the mid-morning one that goes first, so you can start to offer them their snack followed by milk. Gradually reduce the amount they take, but as always, think about your baby's needs and follow their cues.

Naps

No changes with your baby's naps. They will continue to need two for a while longer. A late-afternoon 'danger nap' can cause problems, so try to avoid it as much as possible.

Play

Your baby will now be confidently sitting up, rolling and making good attempts at crawling. They may even be using furniture to pull themselves up. They will react and respond when spoken to and engage in play through noises and facial expressions. You will see a difference in their hand-to-eye co-ordination and the grasping of objects, and start to notice recognition of repetitive words, such as 'hi' and 'bye'.

Some ideas for play include: music and singing, stacking toys, hiding games with toys, ball rolling, messy play with food, talking, playing and reading together.

Sleep

You should be getting more consistently settled nights, with baby going to bed at roughly 6.30/7pm and sleeping through until 6/7am (on a 7am–7pm routine). Although we talk about babies and children sleeping through, they do still progress through sleep cycles. This means when a baby is in a light sleep cycle, they are more likely to become fully awake if the environment alters (e.g. temperature change, room becomes lighter/darker, unexpected noise). Often, during the lighter sleep phase, your baby will become wrigglier and possibly make some noise, too. The key thing here is they are ok and do not need you; it's just like when we roll over in the night and go back to sleep.

Early Waking

Be aware that early rising is most commonly related to overtiredness. With this in mind, ensure your baby is napping enough and going to bed on time. It's good to have a time in your head that is the earliest that you would be happy to start your day. Our advice would be no earlier than 6am. Before this time, treat any wake-ups as overnight time and resettle if required or let baby settle themselves.

Your Question

Q. I am feeding my 9-month-old through the night but I know they (and I) are ready to stop. However, I'm worried about how to go about it. Can you help?

A. Have a look at their day routine – make sure they are getting enough milk and solid food during daylight hours and that their nap times are correct for their needs. Then, when they wake at night, you can feel confident that their nutritional needs have been met and use settling techniques first, rather than milk to get them to go back over. You can go cold turkey at this age (with help from a partner or family member, so they can settle baby) but if you don't want to or it seems too daunting, try to set goals. For example, if you've managed to resettle until 1am one night, you should aim not to feed them the following night until 1am or later, regardless of what they do. Then the next night it might be 2am, and the following 4am and after each new milestone is reached, aim not to feed them until that time. You can also reduce the time they're feeding or quantity, until gradually feeds stop, but this can be hard to gauge. If you feel like they're not taking enough during the day, it is possible they might be overcompensating at night, so in a circular way you need to stop what they're having at night to make sure that they take on more during the day.

You'll find more of your questions in our Troubleshooting Guide (see p. 278).

9-months Routines

Our babies are not robots and you will still have the occasional broken night or disrupted day. And remember, you have half an hour each side to accommodate flexibility – so, if baby was to wake up at 6.30am rather than 7am or sleep until 7.30am, that still works with the same routine.

The following routines are suitable for a baby who is steadily gaining weight and has no medical or feeding issues.

Longer Afternoon Nap

- **7am: awake** Offer milk.
- **7.45am: breakfast** Porridge, cereal, pancakes, toast or an assortment of options.
- **9am: nap** This should be no longer than 30 minutes. If you are putting your baby into their bed at 9 and they are taking longer to get to sleep, push it back to 9.15 or 9.30.
- **10am: snack and then offer milk, if you still are** If they are less interested in milk, it's ok to drop it and offer water instead. Rice cakes, oatcakes, yoghurt are all good snack options.
- **11.45: lunch** If possible, make this a good meal, e.g. spaghetti Bolognese, risotto, lasagne, fish pie, soup with bread. You want to offer lunch before your baby is too tired to ensure they are nice and full ahead of their next nap.

- **12.30: nap** Where possible, this should be at home. This is the nap that your baby will drop last, so it's the longest of the day. It can be up to two-and-a-half hours. If baby wakes before 90 minutes, try to resettle them to ensure they are getting enough sleep across the day. It's also ok to mix things up – so, if one day you are out all day, your baby can sleep wherever you are (buggy, car seat or even the floor).
- **3pm: milk and a small snack** Ideas above. Now is a perfect time to get outside for a nice long walk, meet friends or attend classes. If possible, also allow baby a chance to have a play.
- **4.45pm: dinner** It's a good idea to make things you can all eat to save some time, even if you don't eat together. There will now be time for a play after dinner. High-chair toys are good for this time of day, allowing you an opportunity to tidy up after dinner.
- **6pm: bath time** Using a sitting support can make bath time more fun. Don't fill the bath fully – just enough for a good splash. And don't spend too long in the bath but let them have fun!
- **6.30pm: bedtime** You want to be in your baby's room now getting ready for their last feed of the day. If you are using a sleeping bag, put your baby in it before starting the feed. If using a noise device, start it when you are doing the final wind. Winding is perhaps the most important with this feed, as you don't want baby waking after a short burst of sleep feeling uncomfortable. When you are satisfied baby has finished their milk and is sufficiently winded, it's time for bed. Follow the same routine every night – e.g. kiss, cuddle, into bed, 'night, night', lights off, leave the room.
- **Overnight** Once you have popped your baby into bed and left the room, listen to how they sound, rather than just going straight back in. Try to follow 'Stop, Listen, Look (see

p. 61). If baby looks or sounds like they are just having a grumble, leave them for a little while to see if they settle themselves. If the grumble turns into more of a cry or you feel they are not going to settle by themselves, return to the room and use settling techniques (e.g. if they're sleeping on their back, rub their tummy or head; if they're on their front, pat their bottom). Use these techniques until baby is calm and then leave the room and follow the same guidelines again, if needed.

Longer Morning Nap

- **7am: awake** Offer milk.
- **7.45am: breakfast** Porridge, cereal, pancakes, toast or an assortment of options.
- **9am: nap** This should ideally be two to two-and-a-half hours. If baby wakes before 90 minutes, persevere with resettling. Ideally, you want this nap at home if possible.
- **11.30am: snack and then offer milk, if you still are** If they are less interested in milk, it's ok to drop it and offer water instead. Rice cakes, oatcakes, yoghurt are all good snack options.
- **1.30pm: lunch** If possible, make this a good meal, e.g. spaghetti Bolognese, risotto, lasagne, fish pie, soup with bread. You want to offer lunch before baby is too tired to ensure they are nice and full ahead of their next nap.
- **2.30pm: nap** Your baby will be showing tired signs. Ideally, you want this nap at home if the morning one was on the move. Cap it at 30 minutes.
- **3pm: milk and a small snack** Now is a perfect time to get outside for a nice long walk, meet friends or attend classes. If possible, also allow baby a chance to have a play.

- **4.45pm: dinner** It's a good idea to make things you can all eat to save some time, even if you don't eat together. There will now be time for a play after dinner. High-chair toys are good for this time of day, allowing you an opportunity to tidy up after dinner.
- **6pm: bath time** Using a sitting support can make bath time more fun. Don't fill the bath fully – just enough for a good splash. And don't spend too long in the bath (around 15–20 minutes is fine), but let them have fun!
- **6.30pm: bedtime** You want to be in your baby's room now getting ready for their last feed of the day. If you are using a sleeping bag, put baby in it first. If using a noise device, start it when you are doing the final wind. Winding at this feed is perhaps the most important of all, as you don't want baby waking after a short burst of sleep feeling uncomfortable. When you are satisfied baby has finished their milk and is sufficiently winded, it's time for bed. Follow the same routine every night – e.g. kiss, cuddle, into bed, 'night, night', lights off, leave the room.
- **Overnight** Once you have popped your baby into bed and left the room, listen to how they sound, rather than just going straight back in. Try to follow 'Stop, Listen, Look (see p. 61). If baby looks or sounds like they are just having a grumble, leave them for a while to see if they settle themselves. If the grumble turns into more of a cry or you feel they are not going to settle by themselves, return to the room and use settling techniques (e.g. if they're sleeping on their back, rub their tummy or head; if they're on their front, pat their bottom). Use these techniques until baby is calm and then leave the room and follow the same guidelines again, if needed.

10–12 Months

Crib Notes

- They may be on the move.

- They are likely to have dropped their mid-morning feed, but their routine stays much the same.

- You may need to start saying 'no'.

- If you are struggling with early waking, look back at 'Deal With Early Waking' (see p. 155) for help.

Baby

After so many changes so far in baby's life it will be a relief to know that their routine doesn't change too much in these months. The biggest change will be in them, as they start to push boundaries physically and mentally.

They will now be much more interactive and possibly using furniture to pull themselves up and cruise around, so think about safety and move anything that they may be able to reach and pull down.

You

Day-to-day parenting might feel like it's finally beginning to click into place. You have almost put in your 10,000 hours to be an expert in your baby. This may give you the confidence to get out more and do more things, both with your baby and, possibly, without them.

If your baby is on the move, you may be finessing your ninja skills as you leap across the room to grab the nearest lamp. Again.

Food

Continue offering three good meals a day, increasing lumpiness and texture, as well as two good snacks. Be led by your baby for portion sizes – it's always better for them to finish a plate/bowl of food and then offer more if they seem hungry or ask for it. They will tell you when they are full. Giving them their own bowl and spoon with a small amount in it is a good idea, but you keep one, too, so you know how much they are eating.

It's likely they will now start to show signs of dropping their afternoon milk feed and replacing it with a snack. Offer them their snack and some water followed by milk. Gradually reduce the amount they take, but as always, think about your baby's needs and follow their cues.

Naps

Don't panic – they still need two naps for a little while longer.

Play

You may feel like your little one is starting to push boundaries a bit now. If they are consistently reaching for items or finding things at their level that are not appropriate to play with, you should move baby away and, in a firm, clear but calm voice say, 'No'.

Some ideas for play include: walkers and push-along toys, hiding games with toys, sensory painting and Play-Doh, balls, pop-up or cause-and-effect toys, talking, playing and reading together.

Sleep

You should now be getting more consistently settled nights, with baby going to bed at roughly 6.30/7pm and sleeping through until 6/7am (on a 7am–7pm routine). Although we talk about babies and children sleeping through, they do still progress through sleep cycles; this means when a baby is in a light sleep cycle, they are more likely to become fully awake if the environment alters (e.g. temperature change, room becomes lighter/darker, unexpected noise). Often, during the lighter sleep phase, baby will become wrigglier and possibly make some noise, too. The key thing here is they are ok and do not need you; it's just like when we roll over in the night and go back to sleep.

If your baby becomes fully awake and upset, give them a chance to resettle themselves and if they can't, go in to assist with settling. Try to use hands-on settling techniques and be consistent with your approach. (See the 'No-lift Settle', page 104.)

Early Waking

Remember, early rising is often the result of overtiredness. With this in mind, ensure that baby is napping enough and going to bed on time. It is good to have a time in your head that's the earliest you would be happy to start your day. Our advice would be no earlier than 6am. Before this time, treat any wake-ups as overnight time and resettle if required or let baby settle themselves.

Your Question

Q. My daughter wakes at 5am each morning. We've tried everything and she won't go back to sleep. Then we're all exhausted. Sometimes she will go back to sleep around 7am but then our whole day is out.

A. Early waking is often a sign of something being out in the daytime, so make sure your daughter is following the right routine and that she is having the right number of naps for her age and stage. She may also need more in the way of solids, particularly towards bedtime.

Perhaps something has changed in her environment. Is it coming into summer and getting lighter in her room? If so, look at making it darker in her room – blackout blinds can really help.

If you don't already, you could use white noise or a sleep sound from 4.30am for several nights (some white-noise products come on automatically). This may be enough to get her over the hump (and habit) of waking early.

You'll find more of your questions in our Troubleshooting Guide (see p. 278).

10–12-months Routines

Remember, you have half an hour each side for flexibility – so, if baby was to wake up at 6.30am rather than 7am or sleep until 7.30am, that still works with the same routine. Our babies are not robots, and you will still have the occasional broken night or disrupted day.

The following routines are suitable for a baby who is steadily gaining weight and has no medical or feeding issues.

Longer Afternoon Nap

- **7am: awake** Offer milk.
- **7.45am: breakfast** Porridge, cereal, pancakes, toast or an assortment of options.
- **9am: nap** This should be no longer than 30 minutes. If you are putting your baby into their bed at 9 and they are taking longer to get to sleep, push it back to 9.15 or 9.30.
- **10am: snack** Rice cakes, oatcakes, yoghurt are all good options.
- **12pm: lunch** If possible, make this a good meal, e.g. spaghetti Bolognese, risotto, lasagne, fish pie, soup with bread. You want to offer lunch before baby is too tired to ensure they are nice and full ahead of their next nap.
- **12.30: nap** Where possible, this should be at home. This is the nap that your baby will drop last, so it's the longest of the day. It can be up to two-and-a-half hours. If baby wakes before 90 minutes, try to resettle them to ensure they are getting enough sleep across the day. It's also ok to mix things up – so, if one day you are out all day, baby can sleep wherever you are (buggy, car seat or even the floor).
- **3pm: snack and then offer milk, if you still are** If they are less interested in milk, it's ok to drop it and offer water instead. Now is a perfect time to get outside for a nice long walk, meet friends or attend classes. If possible, also allow baby a chance to have a play.
- **4.45pm: dinner** It's a good idea to make things you can all eat to save some time, even if you don't eat together. There will now be time for a play after dinner. High-chair toys are good for this time of day, allowing you an opportunity to tidy up after dinner.
- **6pm: bath time** Using a sitting support can make bath time more fun. Don't fill the bath fully – just enough for a

good splash. And don't spend too long in the bath, but let them have fun!

- **6.30/6.45pm: bedtime** You want to be in your baby's room now getting ready for their last feed of the day. If you are using a sleeping bag, put baby in it first. If using a noise device, start it when you are doing the final wind. Winding with this feed is perhaps the most important of all, as you don't want baby waking after a short burst of sleep feeling uncomfortable. When you are satisfied baby has finished their milk and is sufficiently winded, it's time for bed. Follow the same routine every night (e.g. kiss, cuddle, into bed, 'night, night', lights off, leave the room).

- **Overnight** Once you have popped your baby into bed and left the room, listen to how they sound, rather than just going straight back in. Try to follow 'Stop, Listen, Look (see p. 61). If baby looks or sounds like they are just having a grumble, leave them for a while to see if they settle themselves. If the grumble turns into more of a cry or you feel they are not going to settle by themselves, return to the room and use settling techniques (e.g. if they're on their back, rub their tummy or head; if they're on their back, pat their bottom). Use these techniques until baby is calm, then leave the room and follow the same guidelines again, if needed.

Longer Morning Nap

- **7am: awake** Offer milk.
- **7.45: breakfast** Porridge, cereal, pancakes, toast or an assortment of options.
- **8.45: snack** Rice cakes, oatcakes, yoghurt are all good options.
- **9/9.15am: nap** This nap should ideally be two to two-and-a-half hours. If your baby wakes before 90 minutes,

persevere with resettling. You want this nap at home, if possible.

- **12.30pm: lunch** If possible, make this a good meal, e.g. spaghetti Bolognese, risotto, lasagne, fish pie, soup with bread. You want to offer lunch before baby is too tired to ensure they are nice and full ahead of their next nap.
- **2.30pm: nap** Baby will be showing tired signs. Ideally, you want this nap to be at home if the morning one was on the move. Make sure it's no longer than 30 minutes.
- **3pm: snack and then offer milk, if you still are** If they are less interested in milk, it's ok to drop it and offer water instead. Now is a perfect time to get outside for a nice long walk, meet friends or attend classes. If possible, also allow baby a chance to have a play.
- **4.45pm: dinner** It's a good idea to make things you can all eat to save some time, even if you don't eat together. There will now be time for a play after dinner. High-chair toys are good for this time of day, allowing you an opportunity to tidy up after dinner.
- **6pm: bath time** Using a sitting support can make bath time more fun. Don't fill the bath fully – just enough for a good splash. And don't spend too long in the bath (around 15–20 minutes is fine), but let them have fun!
- **6.30/6.45pm: bedtime** You want to be in your baby's room now getting ready for their last feed of the day. If you are using a sleeping bag, put baby in it first. If using a noise device, start it when you are doing the final wind. Winding with this feed is perhaps the most important of all, as you don't want baby waking after a short burst of sleep feeling uncomfortable. When you are satisfied baby has finished their milk and is sufficiently winded, it's time for bed. Follow the same routine every night (e.g. kiss, cuddle, into bed, 'night, night', lights off, leave the room).

- **Overnight** Once you have popped baby into bed and left the room, listen to how they sound, rather than just going straight back in. Try to follow 'Stop, Listen, Look (see p. 61). If baby looks or sounds like they are just having a grumble, leave them for a while to see if they settle themselves. If the grumble turns into more of a cry or you feel they are not going to settle by themselves, return to the room and use settling techniques (e.g. if they're sleeping on their back, rub their tummy or head; if they're on their front, pat their bottom). Use these techniques until baby is calm, then leave the room and follow the same guidelines again, if needed.

12–14 Months

Crib Notes

- **Parent party!**
- **You might feel emotional about this milestone.**
- **They will be on the move – and so might be your favourite lamp!**
- **They might be able to follow simple instructions . . . this could be the start of something beautiful!**

Baby

This is such an exciting time for language development. Although baby doesn't always have a lot of words, they are starting to form more conversational babble, and taking it in turns to speak with you. They will be responding to simple instructions, like, 'Give it to Mummy', 'Come to Daddy'. Sadly, it will take them a long time to follow 'Can you tidy your room, please?'

Lots of talking helps language development. This can be as simple as reading whatever article or book you are reading at the time – it does not need to be for children if you don't want it to be. Just listening to your voice and tone is good for them, so it's important you enjoy it, too.

You

Once you reach baby's first birthday, you can start to feel quite emotional looking back at how far you've both come. One minute they're cute, crying potatoes, the next they're little people with strong likes and dislikes (possibly about potatoes).

You may find yourself reliving some of the big events of the last year: their first smile, the first time they babbled your name, the first nappy after they ate blueberries. And if there were any traumas, including the birth, you might find yourself more able to think about them or seek help to address them.

There might be looking back, but there might also be some looking forwards – introducing your baby to different childcare arrangements, returning to work and, perhaps, feeling more ready to spend larger amounts of time away from them. Oh, and the complex matter of whether you should do a birthday-cake smash photoshoot for them.

Food

Solid food is now the main part of your baby's diet. They will still have milk in the morning and at bedtime, but they will also be having three good meals a day and two good snacks. They will now be drinking from a cup and holding a spoon. We would still advise you to have a bowl and a spoon for their food yourself, too, as it can help you to monitor how much food your baby is taking. The food will now be thicker in texture and your baby will be more confident with finger foods.

Naps

Usually between 13 and 16 months your baby will be ready to drop down to just one longer nap, although it can happen as early as 12 months. (It may have happened already if your baby is in childcare.) A lot of parents worry about this change but, as we discussed (see 'Drop Naps Without Losing Sleep', p. 133), it can sometimes be a relief, giving you more time for adventures.

When you are confident that they are ready to drop to one nap, begin by reducing the morning nap right back to 10 minutes and then bring lunch forwards. The next step is to remove the morning nap completely. Do this by bringing lunch forwards to roughly 11am (so they are not overtired) for a short period of time and then their long nap from 11.30/45 for up to two-and-a-half hours. This can be pushed slightly later each day, as they cope with the nap drop, until you get to 12.30/1pm.

Where possible, we recommend that when going through a routine transition, naps are kept at home for at least a week. Prepare the room as you would for bedtime and use the same routine to get them to sleep.

Play

You will be seeing far more control with your little one's movements: going from standing to sitting will be more of a controlled bump and you will see they are pulling themselves up to stand with more purpose. Not all babies will be walking (and might not for some time) but most will be confidently crawling, shuffling, cruising and kneeling. Their engagement with toys and play will also be changing. You will see your baby establishing more of a grasp on smaller objects, toys, crumbs, your skin! They will also follow the movements of smaller toys with their eyes and take more interest in coloured pictures. Some ideas for play include: walkers and push-along toys, hiding games with toys, Play-Doh, sensory painting, balls, standing at doors and windows and interacting, talking, playing and reading together.

Sleep

You should now be getting more consistently settled nights, with your baby going to bed at roughly 6.30/7pm and sleeping through until 6/7am (on a 7am–7pm routine). Although we talk about babies and children sleeping through, they do still progress through sleep cycles – so, when a baby is in a light sleep cycle, they are more likely to become fully awake if the environment alters (e.g. temperature change, room becomes lighter/darker, unexpected noise). Often, during this light sleep, baby will become wrigglier and possibly make some noise, too. The key thing here is they are ok and do not need you; it's just like when we roll over in the night and go back to sleep. If baby becomes fully awake and upset, give them a chance to resettle themselves and if they can't, go in to assist with settling. Try to use hands-on settling techniques in their cot or sleeping space, e.g. shush-pat. Be consistent with your approach.

Your Question

Q. **My baby just had their first birthday but now seems bored of me and always a bit frustrated. Am I doing something wrong?**

A. This can be a confusing developmental stage. They want to do so much more physically and verbally and may be making noises which sound annoyed or frustrated and you can find yourself wondering if you should be doing something differently. However, it is often just a stage of their language development. So, firstly, don't worry – it's not you, it's them; they're just communicating how they feel.Encourage them to try out new skills and think outside the box when it comes to playtime. A bath in the middle of the day can be hugely entertaining, and when you have had enough of entertainment, going for a walk is always a good thing.

You'll find more of your questions in our Troubleshooting Guide (see p. 278).

12–14-months Routines

Our babies are not robots and you will still have the occasional broken night or disrupted day. And remember, you have half an hour each side for flexibility – so, if baby was to wake up at 6.30am rather than 7am or sleep until 7.30am, that still works with the same routine.

The following routines are suitable for a baby who is steadily gaining weight and has no medical or feeding issues.

Longer Afternoon Nap

- **7am: awake** Offer milk.
- **7.45am: breakfast** Porridge, cereal, pancakes, toast or an assortment of options.
- **9am: nap** This should be no longer than 30 minutes. If you are putting your baby to bed at 9 and they are taking longer to get to sleep, push it back to 9.15 or 9.30.
- **10am: snack** Rice cakes, oatcakes, yoghurt are all good options.
- **12pm: lunch** If possible, make this a good meal, e.g. spaghetti Bolognese, risotto, lasagne, fish pie, soup with bread. You want to offer lunch before baby is too tired to ensure they are nice and full ahead of their next nap.
- **12.30pm: nap** Where possible, this should be at home. This is the nap that baby will drop last, so it's the longest of the day and can be up to two-and-a-half hours. If baby

wakes before 90 minutes, try to resettle them to ensure they are getting enough sleep across the day. It's also ok to mix things up – so, if one day you are out all day, baby can sleep wherever you are (buggy, car seat or even the floor).

- **3pm: snack** Rice cakes, oatcakes, yoghurt are all good options. Now is a perfect time to get outside for a nice long walk, meet friends or attend classes. If possible, also allow baby a chance to have a play.
- **4.45pm: dinner** It's a good idea to make things you can all eat to save some time, even if you don't eat together. There will now be time for a play after dinner. High-chair toys are good for this time of day, allowing you an opportunity to tidy up after dinner.
- **6pm: bath time** Using a sitting support can make bath time more fun. Don't fill the bath fully – just enough for a good splash. And don't spend too long in the bath, but let them have fun!
- **6.30pm: bedtime** You want to be in your baby's room now getting ready for their last feed of the day. If you are using a sleeping bag, put baby in it first. If using a noise device, start it when you are doing the final wind. Winding with this feed is perhaps the most important of all, as you don't want baby waking after a short burst of sleep feeling uncomfortable. When you are satisfied your baby has finished their milk and is sufficiently winded, it's time for bed. Follow the same routine every night – e.g. kiss, cuddle, into bed, 'night, night', lights off, leave the room.
- **Overnight** Once you have popped your baby into bed and left the room, listen to how they sound, rather than just going straight back in. Try to follow 'Stop, Listen, Look (see p. 61). If baby looks or sounds like they are just having a grumble, leave them for a while to see if they settle themselves. If the grumble turns into more of a cry or you

feel they are not going to settle by themselves, return to the room and use settling techniques (e.g. if they're sleeping on their back, rub their tummy or head; if they're on their front, pat their bottom). Use these techniques until baby is calm and then leave the room and follow the same guidelines again, if needed.

Longer Morning Nap

- **7am: awake** Offer milk.
- **7.45am: breakfast** Porridge, cereal, pancakes, toast or an assortment of options.
- **9am: nap** This should ideally be two to two-and-a-half hours. If baby wakes before 90 minutes, persevere with resettling. You want this nap at home if possible.
- **11.30am: snack** Rice cakes, oatcakes, yoghurt are all good snack options.
- **1pm: lunch** If possible, make this a good meal, e.g. spaghetti Bolognese, risotto, lasagne, fish pie, soup with bread. You want to offer lunch before your baby is too tired to ensure they are nice and full ahead of their next nap.
- **2.30pm: nap** Your baby will be showing tired signs. Ideally, you want this nap to be at home if the morning one was on the move and cap it at 30 minutes.
- **3pm: milk and a small snack** Now is a perfect time to get outside for a nice long walk, meet friends or attend classes. If possible, also allow baby a chance to have a play.
- **4.45pm: dinner** It's a good idea to make things you can all eat to save some time, even if you don't eat together. There will now be time for a play after dinner. High-chair toys are good for this point in the day, allowing you an opportunity to tidy up after dinner.

- **6pm: bath time** Using a sitting support can make bath time more fun. Don't fill the bath fully – just enough for a good splash. And don't spend too long in the bath (around 15–20 minutes is fine), but let them have fun!
- **6.30pm: bedtime** You want to be in your baby's room now getting ready for their last feed of the day. If you are using a sleeping bag, put baby in it first. If using a noise device, start it when you are doing the final wind. Winding with this feed is perhaps the most important of all, as you don't want baby waking after a short burst of sleep feeling uncomfortable. When you are satisfied baby has finished their milk and is sufficiently winded, it's time for bed. Follow the same routine every night – e.g. kiss, cuddle, into bed, 'night, night', lights off, leave the room.
- **Overnight** Once you have popped your baby into bed and left the room, listen to how they sound, rather than just going straight back in. Try to follow 'Stop, Listen, Look (see p. 61). If baby looks or sounds like they are just having a grumble, leave them for a while to see if they settle themselves. If the grumble turns into more of a cry or you feel they are not going to settle by themselves, return to the room and use settling techniques (e.g. if they're sleeping on their back, rub their tummy or head; if they're on their front, pat their bottom). Use these techniques until baby is calm and then leave the room and follow the same guidelines again, if needed.

PART IV

What Do I Do When . . .?

Troubleshooting Guide: Your Questions Answered

We regularly see parenting advice that is conflicting, and, often, doesn't work in real life. Most people don't have the textbook babies we have all read about. That is why it is important to us that our advice works with real people. We are regularly told that our 'Listener Questions' make parents feel better – not only because of the practical support but because they take away the feeling of being the only one who was wondering exactly the same thing.

Never feel you shouldn't need to ask questions as a parent. It shows you want to learn and make positive changes for your family. Plus, none of us knows exactly what we should be doing all the time. You should see our Google search histories!

This next section is a troubleshooting guide with real questions from real parents who needed help and a little reassurance. Hopefully, they will help to put your mind at rest, too.

Feeding

Q. Should I feed my baby as soon as they wake up?

A. When your baby is very small, they are more likely to sleep right up to the time of a feed; or you could even be waking them in order to stick to your feed timings if they are sleepy or you have been recommended to do so by a healthcare professional. As your baby gets older, they will be able to wake and play or have some quiet time before taking their milk, without it feeling like you are stretching them.

If you are following a routine, aim to keep to your timings, though, and remember the 30 minutes of flexibility you have either side of timings and use that if you need to.

> *From birth to 4–5 months, baby will feed every two to three hours; it then changes to every three to four hours.*

Q. I feel like everything tells me my newborn should be sleeping for 18 hours a day, but, honestly, I feel like they are feeding for 18 hours a day.

A. It can be so difficult to separate everything in your day, as you are responding to your baby in the way you think you should be. But it is important to meet all your baby's needs. And they need to feed and to sleep.

There are no rules for how long each feed should last, but try to make each feed count: look for signs of active feeding and wind well between each offering. If you offer the bottle or breast several times with winding in between, you will be more confident baby is full, meaning you can then focus on healthy sleep habits as well.

Try to remember each baby is different and your baby will also change as they grow. Initially, they may take a long time at each feed; they could also become more efficient at feeding.

Q. I'd like to offer a small bottle at bedtime, so my 8-week-old breastfed baby gets used to taking one. I have no idea how much I should give him?

A. A small top-up at bedtime if they are feeding from you before or afterwards is a good place to start with combination-feeding. If your baby is feeding from you first, start by offering 120ml of either expressed breast milk or formula. You can increase this by 30ml if baby is draining the bottle.

If you want to offer the bottle first because you're worried they will be more unsettled, start by offering 90ml of either expressed breast milk or formula. Doing it this way means you can calm baby afterwards by feeding from you if that is what they are used to.

You can also switch it up, starting with one way and moving on to the other.

When you are offering a top-up, it is a bit of a case of trial and error. Some nights baby will take more and some nights less. You can also do it for as long or as short a time as you feel you or baby needs it.

Q. My 6-month-old baby thinks my milk bar is open 24/7; they feed all night, every night.

A. It's likely they aren't feeding from you all night and that they are using you for comfort instead. That's ok, if you're happy with that, but it can mean that you and your baby aren't getting the rest you need. So, if you feel ready, you can start to stretch out the timings between feeds. To do this, you first need to replace some of those feeds with settling. Stop and listen to the sound they are making. Do you need to go to them? Are they just going between sleep cycles? If you decide they *do* need you, go in and try to settle them in their bed without feeding, using the shush-pat or The Sleep Mums' Shoogle and sleep associations set up at bedtime. Then you can gradually stretch out the time between feeds.

If your baby first feeds at 1am, try to stretch this to 1.30am, then the following night don't feed until that time. Then the following night, try to stretch it again to 2am, and then use that as your benchmark.

For a newborn, the amount of time they can be awake is usually a maximum of 90 minutes. Most of this can be spent feeding; however, you need to keep an eye out for your baby's sleep cues, as an overtired baby can show a lot of the same signs as when they are hungry.

Q. My baby is 7 months and I'm feeling a lot of pressure to stop feeding overnight but I'm not ready.

A. Oh, lovely, that's ok. These stages are there as guidance and definitely not for every parent or every baby. There is no right time to make major changes. The key thing to remember is that when you are ready, you will know – and then it will be a success. If you try to make changes before you are ready, you are more likely to find they don't work.

Try to listen to you and your baby. Only you will know when the time is right. That might be when baby weans themselves or it might be when you feel ready for a full night's sleep and able to work towards getting it.

Q. I think weaning my 6-month-old has made his sleep worse rather than better. Is that a thing?

A. Weaning doesn't happen overnight. If you have only just started, they may not be getting enough solids to meet their needs yet. A combination of finger foods and purées at each mealtime can help to encourage them. Just like in the early days of feeding, they are just learning this new skill. Think about what you're giving them, when and the quantities. You want to make sure your baby isn't too tired for a meal, nor too close to a nap, so that they have time to digest the food in case of any wind.

If you are worried about food allergies or intolerances, talk to a medical professional.

> *Sometimes when babies first start eating food, it can take their digestive systems a wee while to adapt. So, monitoring their poo can help, as can a little leg cycling if baby is a bit constipated. As well as – of course – some prunes!*

Naps

Q. My baby completely refuses to nap. HELP!

A. Naps are not mystical but sometimes it can feel like they are. Firstly, it's really important to make sure your baby is on an age-appropriate routine, getting enough food at the right times of day and that they are going down for naps before they are overtired. That can mean giving them long enough to settle in their bed before the time they should be asleep – this could be as little as a few minutes. Use the same settling techniques as you would at night (see 'Learn How to Settle Your Baby', p. 98).

> *Remember The Sleep Mums' Rule of Three. It will generally take at least three days to instil new nap habits, so stick with it. You'll get there.*

Q. My baby sleeps well at home but I have tried everything, and she just won't sleep in the pram. Is there anything I can do?

A. If they sleep well in their cot or bed, this might not be too much of a problem. Many people find they use the pram to get their baby to sleep, which can be more restrictive. Some children are too distracted by all the light and sounds they encounter in a pram or out for a walk, but others are lulled to sleep by them. You could spend time working on getting baby to sleep in a pram by making it a regular walk (several times a week) at the time of their nap and by making sure the environment is as consistent as possible. You can get snooze shades for prams and buggies that safely block out the light, and use white noise.

If you do manage to get her to sleep and she wakes early, don't rush to stop or lift her. Instead, view it as quiet time – so although she may not be sleeping, she is not being stimulated and still has the opportunity to go back to sleep if she can.

Q. **If my 10-month-old baby's nap gets disrupted, especially the short morning one, what should I do? Can I let her sleep longer? Do I spend the whole nap settling her?**

A. If you are following a 7am–7pm routine, have her awake by 10/10.15am from her first nap. She may not always get the full 30 minutes but that way, you are keeping her routine on track and she will be ready for her longer afternoon nap.

In answer to your second question, yes. Even an entire nap spent settling your baby is better for them than getting up and getting your day out of whack. It's also worth remembering that even just being in her bed with you settling her will give her some rest, away from the hubbub of being up and awake.

Q. **I'm a bit unsure how to play this morning. We had a rough night and a very early wake; we've all been up since 5am. Should I just let my 4-month-old sleep for longer at his first nap to get back on track with the day. So, from 8am until 10am?**

A. Bad nights and early mornings not only feel like they throw your day out, but they can also make your head swim with tiredness. Firstly, take a breath. Don't worry about the whole day – you have plenty of time to get back on track. We recommend breaking the day into more manageable sections: morning, afternoon, bedtime routine and overnight. If you can stretch your timings by small amounts within those, you can still easily fulfil your baby's needs and not disrupt the routine too much. While we give the option of a longer morning nap routine it's better not to switch between routines.

Today, try to push sleep until 8.15/30 if you can. He will be able to last a little longer after his overnight sleep, even after an early wake. Then let him sleep for his usual 45 minutes to an hour. He may look for a feed earlier than 10am, so you can try to stretch him or feed him early as you still have plenty of the day to get back to your usual timings. He may need a top-up feed at 11.15 to help him with the longer lunch-time nap, but before you know it, you're back on track.

Q. **What should I do when I've been settling my 7-month-old baby for their entire afternoon nap time and they fall asleep just before I'm meant to get them up?**

A. Oh, man! It's so frustrating when that happens. But, firstly, take it as a win. You managed to settle them. Remember, too, that while it might not have felt that relaxing for you, time in bed will have been more restful for them than being up and about playing. Plus, you also have the half-hour flexibility for all the timings in our routines. If you are following a 7am–7pm routine, let her sleep for half an hour but aim to get her up by 3.30pm at the latest.

Overnight Sleep

Q. **My 4-week-old is a total party animal at night but then sleeps all day (and I am terrible at sleeping during the day). I'm exhausted and I need help.**

A. Sounds like your baby still has their bags packed from Costa del Pregnancy and is a bit jet-lagged. The best thing to do is choose a rough-day routine and try to follow it, making sure that all day feeds are bright and light and those at night are calm and done in a dimly lit room. Start small by feeding at the right times (a full and content baby will sleep easier than a hungry one) before looking at naps, which can feel a bit overwhelming.

You do need to start waking your baby during the day to get them back on to a normal day and night pattern. We know it seems strange to wake baby up but you want them to be getting as much nutrition as possible during the day, so they don't wake for it at night, and you want them to have their longest spells of sleep at night, so they (and you) can rest properly.

Q. **My 3-month-old has been sleeping so well but I'm being disrupted at night hearing her chew her hands and fight with her swaddle. Is she hungry? Or does this mean she is ready to come out of it?**

A. By the time baby gets to around 3–4 months old, chewing their hands tends to be developmental rather than through hunger. It also doesn't necessarily mean she's ready to lose the swaddle; she could have just found her hands and be exploring them. You could use a transitional swaddle, with one of her arms out, giving her a bit more freedom, while maintaining the security of the swaddle. And if you do it this way and it is a disaster, you can easily go back to a full swaddle for a bit longer.

As babies develop and grow, they can, at times, appear very unsettled but not be fully awake or require anything from you. This is where Stop, Listen, Look (see p. 61) comes in really useful.

This could also be an opportunity, if you're ready, to move her crib away from your bed, so you are less disrupted by her noises.

Q. I feel like my baby should be sleeping through because people keep asking me. Should they?

A. If parents had a minute of Zzzz for every time they are asked if their baby is sleeping through, they would be gifted the world's longest lie-in.

This idea of sleeping though is a sticky one. We all go through periods of sleep and wakefulness on a normal night, but as adults, we turn over and go back to sleep. It can take until around six months for babies' sleep cycles to lengthen and hit the first stage towards more extended sleep. The next stage is them being comfortable in linking sleep cycles together. This is different for different babies. So, while baby may sleep through (with no help from a parent or caregiver) before 6 months, it can take time for them to do so solidly, without any wakefulness or making any sounds whatsoever.

However, if you are ready and you feel like your baby is, too, see 'Learn How to Settle Your Baby' (p. 98) and 'Know How to Wean Your Baby from Night Feeds' (p. 167). These are a starting point for giving you the tools to help your baby sleep for longer stretches.

> *Try not to focus on this idea of sleeping through. It can get competitive. Aim for a restful night for your family – because that will be different for you from the next parent.*

Q. My gorgeous wee bundle was sleeping all night like a total champ, but they've started waking regularly. I don't know why. Is there anything I can do?

A. Usually, when babies start to wake more regularly at night (having been sleeping well), it's because there is something in their day that is no longer working for them. Often this means they need to move on to the next age-appropriate routine (some babies are ready a week or so earlier and some later). Have a look at their naps: do they struggle to get to sleep or are they sleeping too late in the day? And look at their feeds: are they hungrier than they were? Could they be ready to start solids?

> *Often the smallest age-appropriate changes can make a big difference.*

Q. I seriously think my baby has an in-built alarm – for 2am. They wake every night at this time. I know they don't need to be fed.

A. It's not unusual for a baby to continue waking at a time when they were previously fed; they have a milk habit, even though they no longer need that feed. Once you are confident their needs are being met and they're not hungry, use settling techniques (and not a feed). Also know that it's ok to leave baby to have a grumble. They will soon realise sleep is better for them than waking for nothing. Usually, this transition will likely only last a few days – remember The Sleep Mums' Rule of Three (see p. 72): three to five days to make a habit; three to five to lose it.

Q. We have happily and safely co-slept with our 11-month-old baby since they were born but now they're ready (and so are we) to move them into their own bed. But whenever we try, they always end up back in our bed.

A. Once you have made the decision to stop co-sleeping, start at bedtime by putting baby to sleep in your bed on their own. This means they first become comfortable sleeping alone in the place they are used to. Then, after a few nights you can move them to their own room and use our settling techniques to calm them with white noise or a shushing noise playing all night. Then stick to the plan. All night!

Alternatively, some people prefer to start the transition with daytime naps. This way, you can get them used to being in their cot or in their own room before you make the change at night. One of the most important things about a baby's sleep space (after safety) is that it is familiar and feels safe to them.

Q. My baby wakes in the middle of the night for around three hours. I've heard it called a split night, but nothing tells me how to fix it.

A. Check your day routine, as split nights can start because something isn't working in their routine – often naps or bedtime. Once you have one split night, it doesn't need to become a regular event, but it sometimes can if baby gets in the habit of being up at this time.

Think about your settling techniques. If you are going in too quickly to your baby, they may not have had enough time to wake, settle and go back to sleep on their own, or wake and get back to a sleepy state ready for settling. As a result, you are interrupting them, possibly overstimulating them. It may also be that they are at an age when less is more – even a bottom pat feels like playtime. If you feel being in the room settling them is causing overstimulation, leave and return after implementing Stop, Listen, Look (see p. 61).

Settling

Q. We have swaddled our little boy since he was born, and it's worked a dream. He's slept brilliantly but he's getting too big for one now and I'm worried about moving him into a sleeping bag because when we tried, we all had a terrible night.

A. Change can take getting used to – for everyone. It may be that your wee one wasn't ready when you tried before. If you are confident that the time is now (once a baby can roll over, they should no longer be swaddled), the best way to transition is gently and slowly. One arm at a time. So, for the first three nights, try leaving one arm out of the swaddle. Then for the next three, leave the other arm out. After that, try taking the swaddle away completely. Plus, keep The Sleep Mums' Rule of Three in mind: it might take everyone a few days (or nights) to get used to the idea (see p. 72).

Q. **My little one will only settle for me and not my partner. It's flattering, but it's also really tiring as I feel like I don't have any back-up. He's 7 months.**

A. As hard as it is, you need to try to be consistent. So, if your partner starts the process, let them finish it. If your baby knows that by staying awake through your partner's settling, they will get to have you, it's unlikely they will go back to sleep. Although it's tough, try to make sure the person who starts the settle works with baby until they are back to sleep. This is not about not responding to their needs; it's about sharing the load and aiming to be consistent. In the beginning, your partner could wear a jumper that smells of you, which can help your baby settle if they are more used to you.

If you struggle to listen to your baby's tears when your partner is trying to settle them, it may be better for you to go somewhere else and try to busy yourself. It can be so hard to give up control but sometimes, taking yourself out of the situation is the only way to clear your head. As parents, we have a very rational (but sometimes irrational) need to be close to our babies. It's good to let a partner take the burden sometimes, too.

Q. I feel horrible even writing this because of how it makes me feel. I have a friend round who is clearly very upset that I have left my baby to cry for more than two seconds. I am having to pretend that I have come up to him. But I am upstairs in the loo hiding because I know he usually does a few big cries before he goes to sleep. Still, it's making me question myself.

A. Everyone has their own style of parenting and knows their own baby. We should be able to stand by our choices, but sadly, that's not always how it feels.

Often, a baby will have a shout or a grumble before falling asleep naturally by themselves. Sometimes they can even become more upset and distressed when you try to settle them because you are essentially overstimulating them when they want to be asleep.

We believe babies have levels of cries and parents learn to read them best. Plus, generally, it's good to let them have a grumble before rushing to their every sound because they are communicating, and you are listening. That's listening to their needs and learning what their cries are telling you.

Don't worry about what your friends think. You do you.

Q. What can I do if my baby doesn't like any of the settling techniques? They seem to complain when I try any of them.

A. It can take time to find the settling technique that works for your baby.

The first thing to say is that if you are just introducing them, this is a change for them, so they may need a few days to get used to it. It's worth persevering with one that *you* like to see if it was the settling itself – for example, if they're used to being picked up or fed – rather than the technique that they didn't like.

Secondly, less can be more for some. Once your baby gets to a certain age, they can find some settling techniques too stimulating. They may even be telling you that they would like to settle themselves (rubbing their head or face on the sheets, for example). We've even had one baby who liked to bump their head against the edge of the cot a few times before going to sleep!

Finally, some settling techniques can be really difficult to do once your baby is on the move. But because they are wriggling away, that doesn't mean that they don't like it. If they are at the stage of standing in their cot, sometimes just letting them rest their head on your shoulder (rather than trying to get them to lie down and find a spot to pat or rub) can be a good way of calming them until they are ready to be laid down to sleep.

Q. One wee question: what should I do when she isn't well? I feel like all common sense goes out the window because I just want her to be ok and to sleep, so I end up doing anything and everything to make that happen.

A. We all feel like this and often do things when our children are unwell that we wouldn't normally do. But that's totally ok because they're babies, and they need love. However, it's also totally ok because you now know (having read this book) how to get back on track. You have all the tools.

It's easier to have consistency and boundaries when they are well, so don't worry too much. Once you and baby are feeling better and you feel ready, start with your day routine and then progress to overnight. Go back to settling them or allowing them time to settle in their cot or bed. Aim to put back in place all the things you had before to have a happy sleeper once again.

Routine

Q. We try to follow a good routine but often our plans change at the last minute (my partner gets called away) and it throws our whole day out. Then our routine is messed up for days and I don't know how to get things back. What should I do?

A. Take a step back and look at your routine. Consistency is key when you've had a disrupted few days. First, make sure naps and feeds (or meals) happen at the same time. Then move on to night-time, making sure your bedtime routine and settling are consistent. We always say three days to create an unwanted habit; three to five days to reverse it.

Q. I don't know where I'm at on some days, so I feel like I don't read my baby and then get in a pickle.

A. This is where it is great to write things down. When you see it in writing, you can often start to see a pattern emerge – and when you know your baby, you gain confidence. Remember, every day won't be the same. You and your baby won't work like clockwork. The idea of a routine is to give you a rough structure to organise your day, but don't worry if it all goes tits up some days. Tomorrow (or even this afternoon) is as good a place as any to start afresh.

Q. I love your routines – they have given me control back and are so easy to follow. However, I find myself worrying about straying off timings.

A. That's great you are enjoying the routines and they are working but they shouldn't feel tying. It's ok to do your own thing and have wild days out, then get back on track. The beauty of following a routine is that you have flexibility within consistency, and you have the tools to get back on track quickly.

As a guide, follow our 4:3 idea – sticking to your timings for four days out of a week. Try not to have your three 'off-book' days together, but sometimes this is unavoidable.

Q. **We're going on holiday and the thought of it is stressing me out so much, I can't see it being much of a holiday! My baby has been sleeping until 7am but we've got an early-morning flight, so I'm going to have to wake her at 4am. What do I do?**

A. Try to make getting her up the last thing you do before leaving and, ideally, put her into a car seat or similar. She may just go back to sleep. If you are still feeding her overnight, give her a feed when you get her up so that you do not have to do it when you arrive at the airport. If she is not feeding overnight, try to wait until as close to her normal breakfast feed time as possible.

Try to time later milk feeds with take-off and landing, as the sucking helps their ears. If baby has a dummy, this can help in the same way.

If baby doesn't go back to sleep after the early wake-up, you might need to adjust her naps so she doesn't get overtired, which can be hard when you're travelling.

It's worth saying, though, that it's only one day. Baby (and you) will be able to get back on track. Tomorrow is another day (hopefully somewhere lovely), so try to enjoy your holiday.

Break-in-Emergency Chapter – Read When You Need

This shit is hard. It is hard emotionally, it is hard physically and it is hard on relationships and friendships. It is likely you are being hard on yourself, too ('I should have done this'; 'Why didn't I do that?' 'I'm doing this wrong . . .') So, we're here to tell you, even though you might not be able to hear us: you have not done anything wrong. You are doing brilliantly. And every decision you have made – and will make – for your baby is made with love.

> *You can't make mistakes or get it wrong because – no matter what anyone else thinks – you are doing what you are doing because it's working for you and your family in some way. And when it stops working, you can change it.*

It is possible that even reading a book about better baby sleep makes you feel anxious, that you should be doing everything differently. So, we want to reinforce the fact that the guidelines in this book are just that – they are there to guide you, for you to take what you need, not to hold you to account.

When all you need is sleep, it can feel like not doing the things the experts or the entire internet tells you to do is going to make things worse. It's not. The right time to make changes is when it is right for you.

We want you to make a diary entry for two months from now, telling yourself that you're doing a really good job. Seriously. Pop it in now. It will only take a sec. Then, when you get to that day, remember how tough things are just now and you will see how strong you are for making it through.

You might plan to do something, as we often recommend, but in the wee small hours, the best-laid plans fall away as you both struggle to fall asleep. It can be difficult, maybe impossible, to muster the mental strength to do anything apart from what you've already been doing. That is ok. It is always ok. Come back to those plans when you can.

As parents, we tend to spend as much time beating ourselves up as we do looking for socks. And neither is ever fruitful. Each day, there are around 897 decisions to be made for or about your child. That's 897 things you might worry about deciding correctly (or not). And worrying about these things is because you care – but chastising yourself that you're doing it wrong will not help you parent better. It will not empower you to do it differently or better next time. If anything, it's just going to make you feel crap and gradually take away your confidence.

We don't want that to happen. We know we've said it before, but we'll say it again, just in case you weren't listening: you are doing a brilliant job.

So, take a breath. Put this book down and come back to it when you feel ready.

But just before you do . . . we promise you that whatever happens, you will be a better parent next month, and better still next year and in five years – because we are all just learning on the job. Us included.

There is never one right way to parent; but you are the right parent for your child.

Making a Plan – Diary Pages

Keeping a diary can help you to take a closer look at your baby's natural patterns, so that you can read them better and gain confidence in understanding how to meet their needs.

Your Baby's Diary

TIME	MILK	SOLIDS	SLEEP	NOTES

Your Baby's Diary

TIME	MILK	SOLIDS	SLEEP	NOTES

Your Baby's Diary

TIME	MILK	SOLIDS	SLEEP	NOTES

Your Baby's Diary

TIME	MILK	SOLIDS	SLEEP	NOTES

The Sleep Mums, Glossary

Having a baby comes with a whole new language. Not only does your voice leap up a few octaves when you talk to your little one, but suddenly you're throwing words or phrases around – such as white noise and The Sleep Mums' Shoogle – like the parenting boss that you are.

But just in case any of the words we've used – or you've heard – are causing you sleepless nights, here's a run down of the most-used terms when it comes to baby sleep.

Circadian rhythm The approximate 24-hour-clock inside our bodies that co-ordinates the timing of a range of physical and mental functions – like sleep. Sadly, it can't be set like an iPhone.

Colic A term you'll hear people use with the authority of a medical expert (you may even have used it yourself). All it actually means is unexplained crying. Not so helpful to you.

Comforters Can be almost anything that gives comfort to your baby.

Danger nap A nap that takes place dangerously close to bedtime. Usually occurs when you're not looking (and why you will often find Cat singing like a wild woman to her children if they are in the car around 5pm).

Early waking Regularly waking before 6am. As much as we would all love a lie-in, anything after 6am is normal waking (for a 7pm–7am routine). If your baby is consistently waking before 6am, treat it as a night-time wake.

Firm pat or rub When we talk about using a firm pat or rub we are referring to laying your hand on baby securely and confidently. You want baby to be able to feel you and be comforted by you. This also allows you to reduce the firmness as baby settles until it's a light hand that you then remove.

Grumble It's ok for baby to have a grumble and whine; this is not a cry – it's a way of developing language and learning new sounds. A grumbly baby is not distressed and could grumble happily for an extended period of time.

Hangry The irrational anger that shows up when you're hungry. Similar but not to be confused with 'Slangry', when you're so sleepy it makes you mad. This mash up of hunger + anger can affect babies, children and adults alike.

Hor-moan(s) Frustration(s) that occur as a direct result of the horror of hormones. Ignore at your peril.

Jet lag When your circadian rhythm (see above) is out of whack from the light–dark cycle because of rapid travel across places/time zones, such as the womb.

Mama-karma As soon as you say 'My baby has/hasn't done . . .', they go right ahead and do the opposite. Babies are born with perfect timing for maximum embarrassment and inconvenience. It's ok, you'll get them back once they're at school.

Melatonin A hormone produced by the body that helps regulate your circadian rhythm (see above) and, therefore, sleep. Melatonin is normally produced in response to darkness.

Nap A short sleep, usually taken during the day, apart from a person's primary sleep period. A nap may also be referred to as siesta, its name in Spanish (or non-existent, depending on your baby!).

Pink noise A more natural sound blocker than white noise (see below) but with the same effect. It is more likely to be rustling leaves, wind or the sound a train makes as it rumbles along.

Power nap A short doze, usually towards the end of the day, that can help baby through until bedtime. The power nap replaces the third proper nap of the day, usually around 5 months, but can quickly become a danger nap (see above). Less exciting than it sounds.

Silent reflux This is where baby shows all the signs of reflux – unsettled during or after feeds, excessive crying, trouble sleeping, discomfort and/or trouble gaining weight – but without being sick.

Sleep associations Any action or routine that helps your baby fall asleep. Children, and even adults, have sleep associations whether they're aware of them or not.

Sleep cues Signs that your baby is getting tired. Being aware and learning the patterns or behaviours your baby uses means you can try to catch them in the window when they are tired, but not so tired that they will have difficulty falling asleep.

Sleep cycle A progression through different stages of sleep. For an adult, this means five different phases, but there are only two for babies: quiet and active. Most people complete several cycles a night.

Sleep deprivation An amount of sleep that is less than that recommended based on a person's age and health. While traditionally used to refer only to sleep quantity, sleep deprivation can also occur through insufficient quality sleep. Can be used as torture.

Sleep props These generally require somebody to do something for your baby. So, things like rocking or feeding them to sleep. All sleep props are not made equally; some can be useful (until they are not), like a soother or dummy, while others can be really exhausting for you (the newborn twerk, for example).

Sleep triggers Similar to sleep associations but more to do with how your body responds. For example, a dark room triggers melatonin in your body, which makes you feel sleepy and more ready for bed.

Split nights This describes when a baby has an extended wake-up in the middle of the night. This then 'splits' their night in two. It usually occurs after baby wakes and becomes overstimulated, whether by you, their environment or sometimes by themselves (if they are levelling up developmentally). It can be a result of naps or bedtime being out of sync.

Startle (or Moro) reflex The instinct that causes newborns to react as if you just jumped out of a cupboard in a bear mask. They spread their arms wide or stiffen and clench their fists for comfort. It can be alarming at first (and funny, which is one of many parenting paradoxes). It can happen when they are awake and when they are asleep. This is why we recommend swaddling for sleep in the newborn days as it can help them feel less freaked out.

The Sleep Mums' Rule of Three In general it takes three to five days to create a new habit (and three to five days to break one).

The Sleep Mums' Shoogle Place your hand on your baby and rock or move gently from side to side while they are lying in their cot or sleep space. You can shoogle someone to sleep but you can't shoogle them awake. Use firmly to start with, becoming gentler, until your baby is asleep or is calm.

White noise A non-descript sound that's a blend of frequencies – it sounds a bit like radio static – it can be used to block out household sounds, snoring and noisy siblings.

Resources

Support

Pandas Foundation

Is a charity and support service for families and their networks who may be suffering with perinatal mental illness, including prenatal (antenatal) and postnatal depression.

pandasfoundation.org.uk

Helpline number 0808 1961 776

Tommy's

Is a charity organisation that aims to make birth safer. They support parents and families after loss, through pregnancy and during the pre- and postnatal period.

www.tommys.org

Mind

A national mental-health charity, also providing specific information and support about perinatal mental health.

www.mind.org.uk

helpline: 0300 123 3393

The Lullaby Trust

Raises awareness of sudden infant death syndrome (SIDS), provides expert advice on safer sleep for babies and offers emotional support for bereaved families.

www.lullabytrust.org.uk

Cry-Sis
Offers support to parents of crying and sleepless babies.
www.cry-sis.org.uk
helpline: 08451 228 669

Pink Parents
Supports LGBQT parents, step-parents and parents of LGBQT children.
www.pinkparents.org.uk

Home-Start UK
A local community network of trained volunteers and expert support, helping families with young children through challenging times, including perinatal mental health.
www.home-start.org.uk/mental-health

Maternal Mental Health Alliance (MMHA)
A charity with a network of over 100 organisations, ensuring women and families have access to high-quality, comprehensive perinatal mental healthcare.
https://maternalmentalhealthalliance.org/resources/mums
-and-families

Dads Matter UK
Dads Matter UK provides support for dads worried about or suffering from depression, anxiety and post-traumatic stress disorder (PTSD).
www.dadsmatteruk.org

Acknowledgements

We're parents so saying thank you is important to us – well, that's what we tell our kids – and we're so grateful to our village that helped push this baby out!

Thank you to our agents, Lauren Gardner and Paul Moreton at Belle Lomax Moreton, and our editor extraordinaire Lydia Good at Thorsons for your belief in us and occasional hand-holding. You got us here – to the end of the book! – in one piece.

Thank you to the team at HarperCollins; your knowledge, enthusiasm and support felt personal, like we'd had a blether over a cuppa and you had joined us on our mission to help parents get more sleep.

Thank you to Dr Niamh Lynch, Helen Campbell, Claire Willers, Jo Basford, Briony Cullin, Jenny Raymond and Sarah Turner; you have been the best cheerleaders two sleep mamas could hope for.

Thank you to the clients who kept asking when there would be a book (because there needed to be a book!) and for the endless personal recommendations.

Thank you to Oli for literally holding the baby and to that baby, Ever, born the month we got our publishing deal, for being a surprisingly thoughtful writing companion.

Thank you to our listeners, we hope we have given you sleep, but you have given us so much more.

And, finally, without us sounding like total cheese balls, we've always said (from when we planned to do a few podcast episodes) that no matter what happens our friendship is at the heart of everything we do; and both of us are so grateful for that and our mutual love of spaghetti hoops!

Index